THE
LIVER
HEALING
DIET

The MD's Nutritional Plan to Eliminate Toxins, Reverse Fatty Liver Disease and Promote Good Health

Dr. Michelle Lai
MD, MPH

Asha R. Kasaraneni
MSc, RD, LDN, CNSC

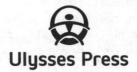

Ulysses Press

Published in the U.S. by:
Ulysses Press
P.O. Box 3440
Berkeley, CA 94703
www.ulyssespress.com

A Hollan Publishing Inc. Concept

ISBN13: 978-1-61243-444-5
Library of Congress Control Number: 2014952009

Printed in Canada by Marquis Book Printing

10 9 8 7 6 5 4 3 2

Acquisitions Editor: Keith Riegert
Project Editor: Alice Riegert
Managing Editor: Claire Chun
Editor: Susan Lang
Proofreader: Lauren Harrison
Index: Sayre Van Young
Front cover design: Matthew Howen
Interior design: what!design @ whatweb.com
Production: Jake Flaherty
Cover artwork: top photo © Steph Stevens, bottom photo © Brian Thompson
Interior artwork: page 3 © GRei/shutterstock.com; page 5 © Alila Medical Media/
    shutterstock.com; page 10 © Designua/shutterstock.com

Distributed by Publishers Group West

NOTE TO READERS: This book has been written and published strictly for informational and educational purposes only. It is not intended to serve as medical advice or to be any form of medical treatment. You should always consult with your physician before altering or changing any aspect of your medical treatment. Do not stop or change any prescription medications without the guidance and advice of your physician. Any use of the information in this book is made on the reader's good judgment and is the reader's sole responsibility. This book is not intended to diagnose or treat any medical condition and is not a substitute for a physician.

This book is independently authored and published and no sponsorship or endorsement of this book by, and no affiliation with, any trademarked brands or other products mentioned within is claimed or suggested. All trademarks that appear in ingredient lists and elsewhere in this book belong to their respective owners and are used here for informational purposes only. The authors and publishers encourage readers to patronize the quality brands mentioned and pictured in this book.

This book is dedicated to Sammi and her soon-to-arrive little sister who have become my biggest motivation for living and staying healthy.
—*Michelle Lai*

To Sriya and her sibling who will be here in a few months. You are the reason why I push myself every day, make good choices, and want to live a healthy, fulfilled life—for the hope that you will also follow your dreams and know that you can do anything you set your mind to!
—*Asha R. Kasaraneni*

TABLE OF CONTENTS

INTRODUCTION

More than 30 million adults in the United States live with chronic liver disease. If you're reading this, you're probably concerned about your own or a loved one's liver health. Whether the problem is mild dysfunction, hepatitis C, non-alcoholic fatty liver disease—or any other liver issues—by opening this book you are on the right path. The first step to a healthy liver is knowledge, and you'll find everything you need to know in these pages.

The most common cause of chronic liver disease in the United States is non-alcoholic fatty liver disease (NAFLD), a condition in which fat is deposited in the liver cells, most often as a result of excess weight. An estimated 30 million Americans have NAFLD, which translates into about 1 of every 4 adults and 1 of every 10 children. Many of these cases go undiagnosed as the vast majority of people with NAFLD do not have symptoms until they develop advanced cirrhosis. This problem is not limited to U.S. borders. There is a worldwide epidemic of non-alcoholic fatty liver disease driven by rising obesity rates globally.

Which leads us to why we wanted to write this book. We met while working together in Boston at Beth Israel Deaconess Medical Center's liver transplant center, caring for patients with chronic liver disease. Michelle is a hepatologist there, working one-on-one with patients who suffer from liver disease as well as researching non-alcoholic fatty liver disease. Asha is a registered dietitian and certified nutrition support clinician specializing in liver health. Between the two of us, we have more than 19 years of hands-on experience in the treatment of liver disease. In all of our years of research and study, we have found that proper nutrition is key to healthy liver function. And so, on a daily basis we counsel our patients on how the liver functions, how it becomes damaged, and how lifestyle changes can make a world of difference to help heal the liver.

While liver dysfunction may seem daunting, there are simple modifications you can make in your daily life to improve your liver's health. In Part 1 of this book, we break down the components of a healthy liver and provide information on liver diseases and dysfunctions. We focus primarily on NAFLD but give you the information you need if you find yourself with a different liver disease or dysfunction. In Part 2, we recognize that the liver is resilient and can repair itself if you detoxify it and move forward with a healthy lifestyle. We share some easy and delicious liver-healthy recipes in Part 3 that will help you implement some of the principles discussed in this book. And in the Appendix, you'll find some helpful worksheets and resources.

The good news is that certain types of liver disease are reversible with a healthier diet, exercise, and weight loss. Early intervention is critical before the damage becomes irreversible. This book will help you on the path to adopting a healthy lifestyle to heal your liver. Here's to a new beginning!

—Michelle and Asha

PART 1

GETTING TO KNOW YOUR LIVER

The liver is one of the most important organs in the body, so keeping it at optimal wellness is fundamental for overall good health. But it's hard to gauge whether your liver is in good shape or not because you can't see it and you can't feel it; it doesn't offer any obvious feedback. When you eat something good, does your liver feel good? When you drink something bad for your liver, like alcohol, does your liver start to hurt? But if you learn a little bit about the liver, you can understand what puts a strain on it and what helps heal it.

In this section, we talk about some of the vital functions of the liver, what the liver does for your body, and the crucial roles it plays in your everyday life. This will help you understand what can go wrong when your liver is sick and injured. Then we detail various liver ailments and disorders—what they are, how they occur, and how you can prevent them.

It's important to understand your liver function in order to see what daily occurrences in your life might be damaging it. So let's have a look.

CHAPTER 1

WHAT DOES YOUR LIVER DO FOR YOU?

A healthy liver is crucial for a healthy life. One of the hardest working organs, the liver performs more than 500 vital functions to keep the body running smoothly. Here are some of the things your liver does:

- Acts as the main food processing system in your body.

- Stores and regulates energy and vital nutrients.

- Breaks down and excretes toxic matter that finds its way into your body through the food you eat and the air you breathe.

- Produces essential proteins that your body uses to function.

In essence, your liver is a processing plant, storage facility, filtering station, and productive factory, all rolled into one. You have only one liver. If your liver is sick and unable to perform its vital functions, the rest of your body cannot work properly. So, just as you carefully maintain your car to keep it running smoothly over time, you need to take good care of your liver so it continues working well. Let's take a closer look at the liver and its functions.

The Anatomy of the Liver

Your liver is located mainly in the upper right area of your abdomen, directly under your diaphragm. It's above your gallbladder, intestines, and pancreas, and above and to the right of your stomach. The liver is connected to the gallbladder and the small intestine by ducts that carry bile. The two main lobes of the liver are made up of thousands of lobules, which consist of liver cells, blood vessels, and bile ducts. Some of the blood vessels carry blood from the heart to bring oxygen to the liver cells and bile ducts. Other vessels carry blood from the intestines to bring nutrients and toxins to the liver for processing. The liver processes and stores the nutrients, and filters the toxins. Other blood vessels carry the detoxified blood away from the liver back to the rest of the body. The liver makes bile, which is carried from the bile ducts to the gallbladder and intestines.

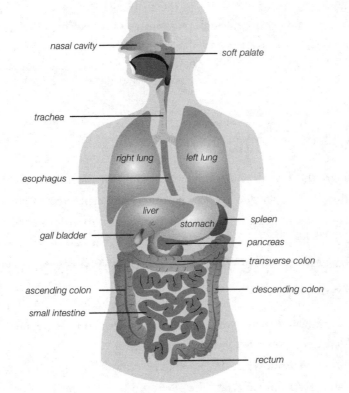

THE ETERNAL LIVER

Did you know that the liver is the only organ in the body that can regenerate itself? The ancient Greeks knew that. In Greek mythology, Prometheus angered Zeus, the supreme god, by stealing fire from the gods and giving it to humans. As punishment, Prometheus was chained to a mountain and subjected to having an eagle eat his liver every day through eternity. The liver would regenerate at night, only to be eaten again the next day.

Other than damage inflicted by a mythological eagle, many other things including viruses, toxins, and diseases can injure the liver. After an injury, the liver will usually regenerate and heal itself. A good example of the liver's incredible ability to regenerate is when someone with a healthy liver donates about half of it to someone with a sick liver. The healthy donor's liver will regenerate to almost its original size in 8 weeks. However, an injuring force that overwhelms the liver's ability to heal or regenerate can lead to severe irreversible liver damage.

Liver Function

Although the liver has hundreds of functions, the four main ones are digestion and absorption of important nutrients; energy storage and regulation; detoxification; and production of important proteins.

Digestion and Absorption of Important Nutrients

Your liver breaks down food into key nutrients such as sugar, fat, and iron, and then helps your body absorb them. It does this by producing bile, which is made from water; bilirubin (a breakdown product from red blood cells); and cholesterol and fat. The bile is produced in the liver, then drained into small bile ducts that drain into larger ones. The bile ultimately flows into the hepatic duct, which then carries the bile to the gallbladder and small intestine. It's here in the small intestine that bile mixes with food to break down fat during digestion. This is important in the absorption of fat-soluble nutrients, such as vitamins A, D, E, and K, which are contained in fat globules. Bile acids break up the fat globules into little droplets so that the vitamins can then be absorbed and utilized.

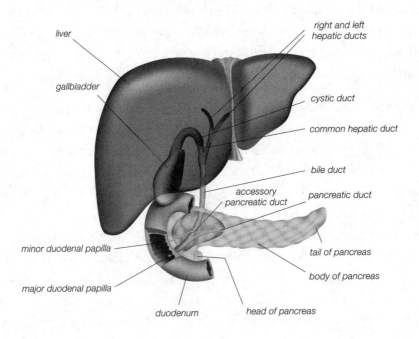

Storage and Regulation of Energy and Nutrients

Think of your liver as a warehouse in which energy is stored and dispensed as your body needs it. It stores and regulates energy in the form of glucose and fructose (the most common forms of sugar consumed in our modern diet). The sugars are stored in the form of glycogen, which is a ready source of energy when your body needs it. The liver can store about 250 to 500 calories of glycogen. It also stores fat; amino acids (components of protein); vitamins A, D, K, and B_{12}; and iron. Exceeding the liver's capacity to store these forms of energy and nutrients can damage the liver. Almost every cell in your body can process glucose as energy. Only liver cells can process fructose. Therefore, excess fructose that overwhelms the liver's ability to process can lead to fat and inflammation in the liver.

Common refined table sugar (sucrose), which most people add to food and use in baking, is half glucose and half fructose. (High fructose corn syrup is 55% fructose and 45% glucose.) After you eat, excess glucose that your body does not immediately use as energy (for walking, running, or all your regular bodily functions) is converted into glycogen for storage in the liver. If you go for a walk after eating, you'll use up some of the glucose you have just consumed so there's less to process into glycogen for storage.

Your liver also takes fructose and immediately converts it to fat to store energy. This is why too much fructose results in fat deposits in your liver, leading to non-alcoholic fatty liver disease (see page 10). When your body needs energy, the liver converts the glycogen back to glucose for energy. If you use up your glycogen store and still need more energy (if you have been fasting or running a marathon), then your liver resorts to stored fat and protein for more energy. Your stored fat is broken down to generate usable energy for your body. Then the liver turns amino acids, which are the building blocks of proteins, into glucose. On the other hand, if you take in a lot more energy that's converted and stored than you use up, the glycogen storage "warehouse" gets overfilled and stops working efficiently.

The liver also processes, stores, and releases iron. When your old red blood cells die, hemoglobin (a protein containing iron) is broken down and the iron is stored in the liver. Iron's role is very important: It helps red blood cells carry oxygen to where it is needed in the body. When the body makes new red blood cells, the liver releases iron to the bone marrow, where it is used to make hemoglobin for new red blood cells. In diseases in which there's too much iron in the body, the extra iron gets deposited in the liver, causing liver damage.

Detoxification

As a fortress that defends your body from toxins, your liver breaks down and eliminates harmful substances. Many of the things you ingest are absorbed in the stomach and intestines, and then into your blood, which flows through the liver to be processed. The liver metabolizes many nutrients, drugs, and poisonous substances that the stomach and intestines absorbed. Harmful substances are broken down into by-products, which are then excreted into the bile or blood. Bile by-products enter the intestine and are eliminated from the body in the form of feces. Blood by-products are filtered out by the kidneys, and eliminated in the form of urine. For example, poisonous ammonia is generated when your body digests protein. It is converted to urea, which is carried through the blood to the kidneys and excreted in the urine.

The liver is vulnerable to reactions and injuries from toxins such as many drugs, including herbal supplements, and excess nutrients (too much fat and sugar) that are processed through the liver. Be sure to check with your doctor before taking any new medications (either prescription or over-the-counter), supplements, or herbs.

In addition to defending your body against toxins, the liver also wards off attacks by bacteria and other infections. Blood from your stomach and intestines flows into your liver and is filtered there. Defense cells in the liver attack bacteria or other infections that may be absorbed by your gastrointestinal tract. Because your liver acts as a filter for blood coming from your stomach and intestines, it is at risk for parasite infections.

Production of Important Proteins

The liver's work is never done. In addition to being a processing plant, a warehouse, and a fortress, it is a constantly operating factory, making vital proteins and cholesterol to keep the body running smoothly.

The liver makes proteins in the blood that transport other important hormones and nutrients to their destinations in the body. For example, it makes albumin, which helps transport thyroid hormone and other hormones, calcium, drugs, and additional molecules around the body to where they are needed. Among the many carrier proteins the liver produces are ceruloplasmin, which transports copper, and transferrin, which transports iron.

The other major role that the liver plays in keeping the body working properly is regulating cholesterol levels in the body. The liver makes cholesterol to export to other cells and also removes cholesterol from the body by converting it to bile salts, which are secreted in the bile and passed from the body in feces. To transport cholesterol and other fats to the rest of the body, the liver synthesizes various lipoproteins (special proteins to transport fat). While we often think of cholesterol as the cholesterol we eat (where too much is bad), the right amount of cholesterol is important for different functions. Cholesterol is a component of the outer coating (membrane) of cells in the body, and it is needed to make bile, which aids digestion. Cholesterol is also needed for the body to make certain hormones such as estrogen and testosterone.

When you stop bleeding after cutting yourself, it is because the liver is doing its job. It makes proteins and other molecules that regulate clotting—both forming blood clots and breaking them down. When there is an injury to a blood vessel, clotting proteins and other molecules work together to make a blood clot that stops the bleeding. Anti-clotting proteins then prevent the blood clot from growing and spreading throughout the body, where it could cause damage by blocking blood flow to where it is needed. When your liver is sick and not able to make these clotting and anti-clotting proteins, you can bleed easily and also form harmful blood clots.

When your liver is sick, you are prone to infections because your immune system is compromised. This is because the liver contains a large number of immune cells and also produces proteins, cells, and other molecules that work to remove bacteria, viruses, parasites, and other foreign bodies from the bloodstream and help fight off infections.

CHAPTER 2

LIVER CONDITIONS & COMMON LAB TESTS

Your liver is like a supermom, multitasking and working constantly to keep the household (your body) running smoothly. When the liver is injured, it cannot do everything it is used to doing, which results in certain nutritional deficiencies. Getting the right nutrients to the liver and avoiding toxic substances so it can heal are crucial. The liver is constantly trying to heal itself, but if the forces that are causing damage overwhelm its ability to heal itself, it will continue to get worse.

You may not have any symptoms while your liver is experiencing ongoing damage, as it will keep working hard, just like a supermom, until it finally wears itself out. Some people with chronic liver disease may have vague symptoms such as fatigue and mild pain in the right upper side of their abdomen. When your liver becomes very sick, you may notice symptoms such as confusion, swelling of your legs and abdomen, bruising and bleeding that occur readily, and jaundice (yellowness of your eyes and skin). Ideally, you want to find out if you have liver disease early on, before the damage is severe and irreversible so that you can get treated and allow your liver to heal.

Liver Disorders

Here are some of the main liver diseases and how they impact the liver and the body. We will discuss how you can contract each illness, what symptoms you may experience, how to prevent the illness, and what the available treatments are for each one.

Non-Alcoholic Fatty Liver Disease (NAFLD) and Non-Alcoholic Steatohepatitis (NASH)

Non-alcoholic fatty liver disease (NAFLD) occurs when fat is deposited in the liver cells as a result of excess weight, diabetes, or metabolic syndrome (high cholesterol, abdominal obesity, diabetes, and high blood pressure).

NAFLD is now the most common cause of chronic liver disease in adults not only in the United States but also in Australia, Asia, and Europe. The cause: an ever-increasing obesity rate worldwide that has created an epidemic of NAFLD.

The most common form of NAFLD is a benign condition called simple steatosis, in which fat accumulates in the liver cells because the liver becomes stressed. It probably does not damage the liver. However, one out of three people with NAFLD has a more serious condition called non-alcoholic steatohepatitis (NASH). Fat buildup in the liver in NASH can cause inflammation and scarring that may lead to severe liver scarring and cirrhosis.

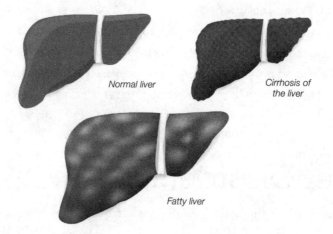

Normal liver

Cirrhosis of the liver

Fatty liver

Being overweight or obese is the usual cause of fat deposits. However, inflammation, damage in the liver, alcohol, and many other factors such as medications and rare diseases can also be culprits. This is why it's important to give your doctor a thorough medical history, including a list of all the prescription medications, over-the-counter medications, herbs, supplements, and vitamins you are taking.

Symptoms

NAFLD usually does not cause symptoms until cirrhosis, liver failure, or liver cancer develops. When symptoms do occur, they can include weakness, weight loss, and pain in the upper right abdomen, Some people might have an enlarged liver felt on physical examination. To diagnose NAFLD and determine the cause and severity of NAFLD, your doctor will do a thorough history, physical exam, and laboratory evaluation, and get an ultrasound of the liver.

Sometimes, a liver biopsy may be needed. A liver biopsy is a procedure in which a small piece of liver tissue is taken to be examined under the microscope for signs of disease or damage. It is most commonly done "percutaneously" by inserting a hollow needle through the skin into the liver. There are currently new tests being developed to assess NAFLD without doing a liver biopsy.

Prevention and Treatment

The best way to prevent NAFLD is to maintain a healthy diet, weight, and lifestyle. Avoid weight gain and get regular exercise.

If you are overweight, obese, or have NAFLD, the best thing you can do for your liver is to lose excess weight and avoid foods high in saturated fat and simple sugar. Fructose, a type of simple sugar, is found in sodas, juices, and many other foods that add refined sugar and high fructose corn syrup. As discussed, your liver converts excess glucose and fructose to glycogen and fat for energy storage. When you take in too much fructose, fat deposits form in the liver and cause fatty liver disease. This fat can then go on to cause inflammation and scarring in your liver. Make every calorie a healthy calorie.

Avoid yo-yo-ing and drastic weight loss because fad diets and starvation techniques leading to rapid weight loss can worsen NAFLD and NASH.

Nutritional Recommendations

- **Lose excess body weight.** Discuss with your doctor the healthy amount of weight you need to lose and a healthy plan for losing it. A good rate of weight loss is 1 pound a week.

- **Lower your intake of simple carbohydrates.** Your liver has to process and store simple carbohydrates (sugars). Excess intake of these sugars puts a strain on your liver. Limit your intake of foods with added sugars.

- **Lower your intake of saturated fat.** Eating a lot of saturated fat can increase the levels of cholesterol in your blood and this increases your risk of developing heart disease and narrowing of your arteries in the body. However your body needs healthy fat in moderation to be able to perform many activities. You will learn more about this later in the book.

- **Increase your intake of omega-3 fatty acids (polyunsaturated fat).** There is some evidence that omega-3s may reduce the amount of fat in the liver. However, the ideal dosage is unknown. Omega-3s are found in oily fish, chia seeds, flaxseeds, canola oil, walnuts, and eggs produced by hens fed greens.

- **Increase your intake of vitamin E.** There is evidence from a clinical trial that getting 800 IU of vitamin E a day can reduce fat and inflammation in the liver for some people with NASH, the more severe form of NAFLD. Roughly half the subjects in this study who received vitamin E improved, but half did not. This study was done on patients without diabetes. Before starting vitamin E, talk to your doctor about whether this is a good plan for you and about any potential long-term risks.

- **Increase your intake of vitamin D.** Vitamin D deficiency is common in patients with NAFLD, as it is in all patients with chronic liver disease. Talk to your doctor about checking for vitamin D deficiency and whether you need supplements.

- **Increase potassium-rich foods.** A study shows a link between low potassium levels in the blood and increased risk of non-alcoholic fatty liver disease. People with liver disease have lower total body potassium stores. A diet high in potassium lowers blood pressure (which then lowers the risk of strokes and heart disease), protects the bones, and reduces the risk of kidney stones. Fruits and vegetables are high in potassium; for more about potassium-rich foods, see Chapter 3. Ideally, your diet should provide at least 4,700 mg of potassium a day. Unfortunately, the average male in the United States takes in 3,200 mg a day, and the average female only 2,400 mg a day. If you are on diuretics (pills that make you urinate and decrease potassium in the blood), then your doctor should monitor your potassium level closely. Ask your doctor how much potassium you should take in daily.

Alcoholic Liver Disease

When your system takes in too much alcohol, your liver can become inflamed and damaged. This is because most of the alcohol that you consume is processed by the liver, detoxified, and broken down into by-products. When you take in too much, these by-products can damage your liver. Although the exact mechanism is not clear, we know that excess alcohol can cause fat production, inflammation, and death of liver cells. This leads to scarring in the liver and, if left untreated, can lead to cirrhosis.

Alcohol-related liver injury can cause deficiencies of the following micronutrients: folate, B1 (thiamine), B3 (niacin), B6 (pyridoxine), B12 (cyanocobalamin), vitamin C, vitamin A, vitamin D, vitamin E, vitamin K, magnesium, and selenium. Some of the deficiencies are caused by poor intake of the micronutrients, if alcohol is replacing other foods as a source of calories. Other deficiencies are from alcohol impairing the liver's ability to absorb, store, and process the nutrients.

Symptoms

Some people may not show symptoms of ongoing liver damage from alcohol. Severe inflammation in the liver, called alcoholic hepatitis, can have symptoms such as loss of appetite, nausea, vomiting, and abdominal pain. In severe cases, there can be swelling of the abdomen, confusion, and yellowing of the skin and eyes.

Prevention and Treatment

The best way to prevent alcoholic liver disease is simply to avoid excessive consumption of alcohol. If you have a different liver disease, you should avoid drinking altogether.

If you already have alcoholic liver disease, the most important thing you can do for your liver is to stop drinking alcohol so that your liver can recover and regenerate itself. Talk to your doctor about which extra nutrients you may need. If your liver is affected by alcohol, your doctor may recommend taking folate, thiamine, and a multivitamin. Keep in mind that the best way to get these nutrients is from food, and most are readily available in fruits, vegetables, and nuts. It is crucial to have a variety of these foods in your diet on a daily basis. If you also have had alcoholic hepatitis (severe liver inflammation from alcohol), your liver will need protein and calories to regenerate. Malnutrition will keep your liver from recovering.

Nutritional Recommendations

• Avoid alcohol.

• Take folate, thiamine, and a multivitamin.

• Talk to your doctor and a registered dietitian to find out what your daily protein and calorie needs are.

Hepatitis A

Hepatitis A is a virus that replicates itself in the liver. It is usually spread by contaminated food or water, or through close contact with an infected person. The virus is shed by an infected person in the feces, which in poor hygiene conditions can contaminate food or water, infecting anyone who ingests the food or water. The hepatitis A virus causes acute liver infection. In trying to kill the virus, the body's immune system ends up attacking the liver cells that contain the hepatitis A, causing inflammation and cell death.

Symptoms

Symptoms of acute hepatitis A infection can include fatigue, jaundice, nausea, vomiting, loss of appetite, discomfort in your abdomen, and light-colored stools. Most people who are infected recover completely without any liver damage. In rare cases, infection can result in liver failure and liver transplantation or death. If you have a chronic liver disease, then you have a higher risk of not recovering from hepatitis A infection.

Prevention and Treatment

Fortunately, there is an effective vaccine against hepatitis A. It is recommended for all children at age 1 and also for people with chronic liver disease or traveling to countries where hepatitis A is common. To see if hepatitis A vaccination is recommended for the countries you are traveling to, go to cdc.gov/travel; enter the countries you are traveling to and the website will tell you which vaccinations (including hepatitis A, if applicable), are recommended. The vaccination requires two shots 6 months apart, but getting the first shot before your travel will still give you some protection.

It is also important to practice good hygiene, especially when traveling to places with poor sanitation. When traveling abroad, take precautions: Wash your hands frequently, avoid uncooked foods, and drink bottled water instead of tap water. Often, ice is made from tap water, so skip the ice in your drink. If soap and water are not readily available, use a hand sanitizer. Eat fresh fruits and vegetables only if you peel them yourself. Otherwise, avoid fruits, vegetables, salads, and raw meat or shellfish in places of poor sanitation. Stick with cooked foods and eat them while they're still hot. Avoid food from street vendors, who often do not have appropriate facilities for proper frequent hand washing and cleaning.

The treatment for acute hepatitis A infection is supportive care: giving intravenous fluids for dehydration and treating the symptoms. If acute hepatitis A infection results in liver failure, the only treatment is a liver transplant.

Hepatitis B

Hepatitis B is another virus that replicates itself in the liver cells. The body's immune system can damage liver cells while trying to kill the virus. Hepatitis B is usually spread through infected blood, semen, or other bodily fluids. Acute infection occurs within the first 6 months after someone is exposed. It can lead to chronic infection, a long-term disease in which the virus lives and multiplies in the liver. The younger you are at the time of exposure, the higher the chance that this will become a chronic infection. For example, the majority of people who were infected with the virus at birth (passed from infected mother to baby) will have chronic hepatitis B infection, whereas only a minority of people exposed to hepatitis B as adults will progress to chronic infection. Chronic infection can lead to severe diseases such as cirrhosis, liver failure, and liver cancer.

The hepatitis B virus is considered a carcinogen (cancer-causing agent). Data from countries where hepatitis B is prevalent have shown a decrease in the incidence of liver cancer after universal vaccination (of all children) against hepatitis B. Suppressing the virus is likely to decrease the risk of liver cancer.

Symptoms

Symptoms of acute hepatitis B infection can range from no symptoms to nausea, vomiting, loss of appetite, mild fever, body aches, jaundice, and liver failure. Most people with chronic hepatitis B infection do not have any symptoms until they develop advanced disease (cirrhosis, liver failure, or liver cancer).

Prevention and Treatment

It is important to be screened for hepatitis B if any of the following risk factors applies to you. Talk to your doctor about screening if you:

- Or your parents were born in a country with a high rate of hepatitis B infection, or you lived in the same household or had sexual contact with someone born in a part of the world with a high rate of hepatitis B, including:

  o Asia

  o Africa

  o South Pacific Islands

  o Middle East (except Cyprus and Israel)

  o European Mediterranean: Malta and Spain

  o South America: Ecuador, Guyana, Suriname, Venezuela, and Amazon regions of Bolivia, Brazil, Colombia, and Peru

  o The Arctic (indigenous populations of Alaska, Canada, and Greenland)

  o Eastern Europe: All countries except Hungary (Hungary has a lower prevalence of hepatitis B than the rest of Eastern Europe)

  o Caribbean: Antigua and Barbuda, Dominica, Granada, Haiti, Jamaica, St. Kitts and Nevis, St. Lucia, and Turks and Caicos

  o Central America: Guatemala and Honduras

- Have ever injected recreational drugs.

- Have had multiple sexual partners or have had a sexually transmitted disease.

- Are a man who has had sex with men.

- Were ever an inmate at a correctional facility.

- Are infected with hepatitis C or HIV.

- Are undergoing renal dialysis.

- Are pregnant.

- Are getting a treatment that lowers your immune system.

There is an effective vaccine to protect you from hepatitis B infection. If you have not been vaccinated, talk to your doctor about getting the vaccine.

If you have chronic hepatitis B infection, see a liver specialist to discuss whether you should be treated or undergo regular ultrasounds to screen for liver cancer.

Nutritional Recommendations

- Avoid foods that might be contaminated with aflatoxins (see page 59).

- As with all chronic liver diseases, vitamin D deficiency is common. Talk to your doctor about whether you should have your vitamin D level checked and whether you need to be on a vitamin D supplement.

Hepatitis C

About 3.2 million Americans have chronic hepatitis C, one of the most common causes of chronic liver diseases. The virus infects the liver, causing inflammation. Over years, it causes damage that may ultimately lead to cirrhosis.

Symptoms

Most people chronically infected do not have any symptoms until they develop cirrhosis and liver failure, so it is important to get screened. Your doctor will order a simple blood test to see if you are infected.

Prevention and Treatment

There is no vaccine against hepatitis C yet. The best way to minimize infection is to avoid sharing needles or razors with other people. You should get tested for hepatitis C if any of the following applies to you. Talk to your doctor about testing if you:

- Were born between 1945 and 1965.

- Received blood transfusions, blood products, or organ transplants before 1992.

- Are infected with HIV (human immunodeficiency virus).

- Were exposed to hepatitis C–positive blood through needle sticks, sharps (such as on scalpels or knives), or contact of the infected blood with your mucous membrane (such as eyes, mouth, and nose) while at work as a healthcare, medical emergency, or public safety worker.

- Ever injected recreational drugs.

There are highly effective treatments to cure hepatitis C. Sometimes people avoid treatment because they've heard that it causes terrible side effects. Previous treatments did include an injection medication and often came with severe side effects that were difficult to tolerate, but that's not the case with newer treatments. Talk to your doctor about treatment options.

Keep in mind that alcohol and hepatitis C do not mix. Alcohol worsens liver damage. Obesity is also known to aggravate hepatitis C infection. It is important to avoid alcohol intake and lose excess weight to help protect your liver from further injury. Vitamin D deficiency is common in patients with chronic hepatitis C, as it is in all patients with chronic liver diseases. Talk to your doctor about testing for vitamin D deficiency and whether you need supplements.

Nutritional Recommendations

• Avoid excess weight gain.

• Avoid alcohol.

• Take a vitamin D supplement if you are deficient in vitamin D.

Cholestatic Liver Diseases

Liver diseases that cause cholestasis, a condition in which your bile does not flow normally, include primary biliary cirrhosis (PBC) and primary sclerosing cholangitis (PSC). Certain infections and reactions to medications can also cause cholestasis.

Symptoms

Some common symptoms are itching and fatigue. In cholestatic liver diseases, the bile is not being excreted and passed out through your gut. The bile acids get backed up into your bloodstream and build up in your skin, causing itchiness. When your bile does not flow normally, your body is unable to absorb fat properly. This leads to high cholesterol and also deficiencies in fat-soluble vitamins (A, D, E, and K). Vitamin D is responsible for calcium absorption, so a deficiency in vitamin D leads to a deficiency in calcium as well. Vitamin D and calcium deficiencies put you at risk for osteopenia or osteoporosis (low bone density), which in turn put you at risk for bone fractures. Osteoporosis is twice as common in patients with PBC compared with the general population.

Prevention and Treatment

Unfortunately, there is no known way to prevent cholestasis liver diseases. Treatment will depend on your specific condition and situation, but often those affected are prescribed a medication called ursodeoxycholic acid (also called ursodiol), a synthetic form of bile acids.

Nutritional Recommendations

- **Get plenty of calcium and vitamin D.** Good intake of calcium (minimum 1,000 mg/day) and vitamin D (at least 800 IU/day) is important to prevent bone loss. If you already have signs of osteoporosis based on laboratory tests, you will prescribed higher doses.

- **Get the proper amount of vitamin A.** The most common fat-soluble vitamin deficiency in patients with PBC is vitamin A. However, too much vitamin A is toxic to the liver. It's best to have your vitamin A levels checked and corrected based on symptoms of vitamin A deficiency, such as night blindness.

- **Take vitamin K supplements if necessary.** If you are deficient in vitamin K, your doctor will recommend supplementation based on your test results and medications you're taking.

Drug-Induced Liver Injury

Because often your liver is the first line of defense, it is prone to injury by various substances including prescription medications, over-the-counter medications, herbs, supplements, hormones, vitamins, recreational drugs, and toxins in the environment (such as aflatoxin, pesticides, and arsenic). Dietary and herbal supplements are less regulated by the government than prescription and over-the-counter medications, and therefore are not required to have the same level of safety evidence of quality testing. There is a misconception that because something is an herbal or dietary supplement, it is harmless. Over the past decade, there has been a rise in liver injury from herbs and supplements, with some of these cases resulting in death or liver transplants.

Symptoms

One sign of drug-induced liver injury is abnormal liver enzymes from inflammation and malfunction of the liver. The symptoms can vary but may include fatigue, loss of appetite, nausea, vague abdominal pain, jaundice, easy bruising, or itchiness. In most cases, your liver will heal itself after stopping the harmful agent. However, the injury can be severe, resulting in liver failure and death or the need for a liver transplant.

Prevention and Treatment

The best way to prevent drug-induced liver injury is to avoid unnecessary medications, herbs, and supplements. Check with your doctor before starting anything new.

If you have drug-induced liver injury, you need to be monitored by your doctor closely to make sure your liver is recovering. Your doctor may give you a course of prednisone to calm the inflammation in the liver. As with any liver injury, you want to make sure you are getting adequate protein and calories to allow your liver to regenerate and heal. Some drug-induced liver injury can result in cholestasis (page 20).

Nutritional Recommendations

• Avoid any unnecessary herbs, supplements, or vitamins.

Iron Overload/Hereditary Hemochromatosis

The liver stores and transports iron needed by the body. Too much iron can damage the liver and lead to cirrhosis, liver failure, or liver cancer. The two most common causes of excess iron in the body are hereditary hemochromatosis and too many blood transfusions. Hereditary hemochromatosis is a genetic disease in which the person absorbs too much iron from the intestines. The iron then builds up in the body, damaging the liver, heart, pancreas, and other organs.

You can also have excess iron from receiving too many blood transfusions. This usually occurs in people with a blood disorder that causes them to have chronic anemia (low red blood cell count), such as thalassemia, sickle cell disease, aplastic anemia, or myelodysplastic syndrome. Thalassemia and sickle cell disease are diseases of abnormal red blood cells. Aplastic anemia and myelodysplastic syndrome occur when the bone marrow is unable to make enough red blood cells. Because red blood cells contain a lot of iron, frequent blood transfusions cause iron to build up in the system and accumulate in the organs.

Symptoms

Many people have no symptoms in the early stages of iron overload. As the disease becomes more advanced, an affected person can develop joint pain, diabetes, or heart failure.

Prevention and Treatment

Once diagnosed, excess iron is easily treated with therapeutic phlebotomy (bloodletting). Your red blood cells carry a lot of iron, so eliminating some red blood cells on a regular basis gets rid of the excess iron. The key is early diagnosis to prevent any organ damage. If you have been diagnosed with hereditary hemochromatosis, make sure your family members are aware so that they can be screened.

If you are not able to tolerate phlebotomy, the alternative treatment is iron-chelating medication, which binds to the iron and helps the body get rid of excess iron.

Nutritional Recommendations

- Avoid iron supplements.

- Avoid vitamins that contain iron.

- Avoid vitamin C supplements (vitamin C promotes absorption of iron).

- Avoid raw seafood (it may contain bacteria that grow well in an iron-rich environment).

Autoimmune Hepatitis

A chronic disease in which the immune system attacks the liver, autoimmune hepatitis causes inflammation and scarring. If untreated, it can progress to cirrhosis and liver failure. The body's immune system normally attacks bacteria, viruses, parasites, and other foreign substances, but in the case of autoimmune hepatitis it mistakenly recognizes the liver as a foreign body and mounts an attack against it.

Symptoms

Symptoms of autoimmune hepatitis include fatigue, itchiness, joint pains, abdominal discomfort, nausea, vomiting, loss of appetite, jaundice, and rashes.

Prevention and Treatment

There is no known way to prevent autoimmune hepatitis. The treatment is medication to suppress the immune system and calm down the inflammation. As with other conditions in which the liver is inflamed, people with autoimmune hepatitis are prone to vitamin D deficiency. One commonly used medication to suppress the immune system is prednisone, a steroid hormone that can put you at risk of osteoporosis. Vitamin D is important for bone health, so it is especially important for people with autoimmune hepatitis on prednisone to get enough vitamin D. Talk to your doctor about testing your vitamin D level.

Nutritional Recommendations

- Take a vitamin D supplement if you are deficient. Talk to your doctor about what dose you should be taking.

- Get plenty of calcium in your diet. The daily requirement depends on age and sex, but generally the minimum amount is between 1,000 and 1,200 mg per day. If you aren't making your quota from diet alone, take a calcium supplement. Vitamin D is important for the absorption of the calcium, so that's another good reason to be sure you get enough vitamin D as well.

Wilson's Disease

Wilson's disease is a rare genetic disorder in which too much copper accumulates in the brain, liver, and other organs, causing damage. If you have been diagnosed with the disease, let your family members know so they can be screened. Diagnosis is made using a combination of blood tests, urine tests, eye exam, and often a liver biopsy. The key is early diagnosis so that treatment can prevent organ damage.

Symptoms

Some patients may not have symptoms early on, but others may experience fatigue, lack of appetite, abdominal discomfort, jaundice, uncontrolled movements or muscle stiffness, or problems with speech, swallowing, or coordination.

Prevention and Treatment

If you have Wilson's disease, you want to avoid food high in copper, such as seafood, mushrooms, seeds, nuts, and dried fruits. Treatment involves taking a medication that binds to copper so that your body can get rid of excess copper.

Nutritional Recommendations

- Use a water filter. Copper is found in drinking water, most often from corrosion of copper-containing water pipes that carry the water.

- Avoid cooking with copper pots. Copper from unlined copper cookware, or from cooper cookware in which the lining has broken down, will leach into food.

Decompensated Cirrhosis

Any chronic liver disease can lead to cirrhosis. Decompensated cirrhosis means that the liver is no longer able to compensate for damage and can no longer carry out all of its necessary functions.

Cirrhosis causes the body to reach a catabolic state, which means that the body breaks down proteins and tissues instead of building and repairing them. This results in muscle wasting, poor healing, and an impaired immune system. Increase calories from protein to slow down the wasting process.

Symptoms

Signs of liver decompensation include fluid in the belly, swelling of the legs, bleeding from distended veins in the gastrointestinal tract, confusion, and jaundice.

Prevention and Treatment

Early diagnosis and treatment of chronic liver disease is the best way to prevent progression to cirrhosis.

Because symptoms may include fluid in the belly and swelling of the legs, a low-sodium diet is essential. Salty foods make the body retain fluid. While your doctor may prescribe medications to help you get rid of the fluid, it is still important to restrict sodium intake.

It's also important to control the belly fluid, which is not only uncomfortable but also responsible for a lot of the muscle wasting seen in decompensated liver disease. Because the fluid makes you feel full, the result is decreased appetite. You use a lot of energy (calories) to keep the fluid at body temperature, and to keep up with this energy demand, your body breaks down muscles.

In general, the recommendation is to consume around 1,500 mg of sodium per day, which amounts to less than 1 teaspoon. Check with your dietitian about specific recommendations.

People with cirrhosis have low potassium stores in their bodies. If you are taking a diuretic (medication to make you urinate), your blood can have a high or low level of potassium, a situation that your doctor should monitor closely. The most common diuretics used in people with decompensated cirrhosis who have belly fluid or swollen legs are furosemide and spironolactone. Furosemide can lower potassium by causing the kidneys to get rid of it. Spironolactone is a potassium-sparing diuretic, meaning that it prevents the kidneys from getting rid of the potassium. Often, people with belly fluid or swollen legs are given a combination of furosemide and spironolactone to balance the blood potassium concentration.

If you have cirrhosis, avoid taking iron supplements unless specifically recommended by your doctor as excess iron can cause further damage to your liver.

As we mentioned, people with cirrhosis can lose protein mass. It is important to get enough calories from protein to slow down the muscle wasting.

People who develop decompensated cirrhosis may eventually require a liver transplant.

Nutritional Recommendations

- **Include more protein in your diet.** The exact amount needed varies greatly from person to person, especially in liver disease patients. Your requirement could be anywhere between 60 and 150 grams per day. Consult with a registered dietitian for the amount that you need. In the meantime, choose healthy sources of protein, such as Greek yogurt and grilled or baked chicken.

- **Cut out salt.** See Eliminate High-Sodium Foods on page 50 for advice on how to cut out excess sodium from your diet.

- **Be aware of your potassium level.** Check with your doctor about whether you should be consuming foods high in potassium.

- **Increase calories.** If you have uncontrolled belly fluid, make sure to get enough protein and calories to meet your needs. Meet with a registered dietitian to discuss your daily protein and calorie needs.

Common Laboratory Tests

These are some of the tests your doctor might order if he or she suspects you have liver disease. All of them require a simple blood draw.

ALT and AST Liver Enzymes

Alanine aminotransferase, or ALT (also known as serum glutamate-pyruvate transaminase, or SGPT) and aspartate aminotransferase, or AST, (also known as serum glutamic oxaloacetic transaminase, or SGOT) are enzymes common in liver cells. Both of these enzymes can also be found in smaller amounts elsewhere in the body—in the muscles, heart, kidneys, pancreas, and red blood cells. When liver cells are damaged or inflamed, they release ALT and AST into the bloodstream, raising the levels of those enzymes. The ratio of ALT to AST can give clues about the cause or severity of liver damage.

For example, the level of AST may be higher than that of ALT in alcoholic liver disease or cirrhosis. Although different laboratories use slightly different "normal" values, most consider an ALT or AST value of greater than 40 IU/L (international units per liter) abnormal. However, a high normal ALT or AST reading can still indicate inflammation in the liver, which in recent years has led to revised abnormal ranges for certain diseases such as hepatitis B, in which the new normal cutoff is now 30 IU/L for men and 19 IU/L for women.

Because these enzymes are also made in other parts of the body, ALT and AST can be elevated from non-liver-related causes. For example, if you did a lot of heavy weightlifting a couple of days before the blood tests, your ALT and AST values may be elevated because the enzymes were released by the muscles. There is more release of AST than ALT from muscles, so your AST value would be higher than your ALT. However, AST breaks down at a faster rate in the blood, so if your blood were drawn a few days after strenuous exercise or muscle injury, then the AST and ALT levels might be about the same.

Alkaline Phosphatase

Alkaline phosphatase is a enzyme whose function is to alter different molecules in the body. It is made in the liver as well as in the bones, placenta, intestines, and kidneys. An elevated level can indicate liver damage or blocked bile ducts. The level can also be high during pregnancy or as a result of bone disease. In Wilson's disease, a genetic disorder affecting the liver, the level of alkaline phosphatase may be low. The normal range for alkaline phosphatase varies from laboratory to laboratory.

Bilirubin

Bilirubin is a substance produced when the liver breaks down old red blood cells. Indirect (or unconjugated) bilirubin is fat-soluble. The liver coverts indirect bilirubin into direct (or conjugated) bilirubin, which is water-soluble. Direct bilirubin is then excreted through the bile to the intestines and finally in the stools. It's a brownish yellow substance that gives stools their normal color. Tests for this substance generally will show the total amount (combination of direct and indirect bilirubin), but your doctor may ask the lab to check the breakdown of both indirect and direct bilirubin levels.

If the liver is not working well and the liver cells are unable to move bilirubin into the bile to pass in the stools, direct bilirubin can build up in the bloodstream, causing the skin and whites of the eyes to become yellow (jaundice). The lab test looks for an elevated level of direct bilirubin, which indicates liver dysfunction, but in some cases the level of indirect bilirubin is elevated. An elevated level of indirect bilirubin could indicate a common benign inherited condition called Gilbert syndrome, in which the liver has trouble turning indirect bilirubin into direct bilirubin. It is a benign condition but does cause some jaundice, especially during times of stress, fasting, or infections. Gilbert syndrome is found in about 5% of the general population.

Albumin

An important protein made by the liver, albumin circulates throughout the bloodstream. The level of albumin in the blood is one indicator of how well the liver is functioning. The normal range is usually around 3.5 to 5.2 (grams/deciliters). When the liver is damaged and not working well, the level of albumin can be low. However, other conditions can cause a low albumin level. If your level is low, your doctor will need to investigate further to figure out whether the cause is poor liver function or some other condition.

Blood Coagulation

The liver produces clotting factors that help stop bleeding after a cut or injury. Underproduction of these factors signals how well—or how poorly—the liver is functioning. The prothrombin time (PT) is the amount of time it takes blood to clot. Because there are variations in PT values among labs, the international normalized ratio (INR) was devised to standardize PT results. If the liver is not working well and not making enough clotting factor, then the prothrombin time will be longer than normal, giving a higher INR. The normal INR range is usually 0.8 to 1.2.

PART 2

TAKING CARE OF YOUR LIVER

Knowledge is power. The more you know, the more you can take control of your health. Now that you know more about your liver, what it does, and what can damage it, let's pivot to what you need to know to care for your liver and get it healthy. First, you'll get a primer on the different nutrients found in foods. It's important to realize which nutrients you might be getting too much of, or too little of, in your diet. Making sure that you get the right amount of each nutrient means knowing how to control portion sizes and how to read labels so you can decipher the nutritional content of foods.

Once you have a good grasp of nutrition, you'll get to the *action* part of the book. That's all about the steps you can take to care for your liver: Eliminate toxins, eat a healthy diet, and reap the benefits of exercise.

CHAPTER 3

NUTRITION 101

To prepare you for your journey to a healthier liver and a healthier you, we have provided this primer so that you know what is nutritious and safe for your body. This chapter starts off with information on macronutrients and micronutrients (and the foods that contain each nutrient), followed by sections on healthy portion sizes and food labels.

We don't expect people to keep track of the amount of each nutrient contained in the foods they eat. The easiest way to get the complete set of nutrients your body needs is to eat a variety of foods daily. Your daily intake should consist of at least 6 to 7 servings of fruits and vegetables, 5 servings of complex carbohydrates, 3 servings of protein, and 3 servings of dairy products. Load up on different colored fruits and vegetables. The reason you want to eat a "rainbow" of fruits and vegetables is that the various colors contain different nutrients.

Macronutrients

Food contains three macronutrients that give our bodies the energy they need to function: carbohydrate, protein, and fat.

Carbohydrate

This macronutrient is the preferred source of energy for the brain, heart, and central nervous system, but it has limited capacity to meet the body's demands beyond a few hours. The three types of carbohydrate are sugar, starch, and fiber. Starch (complex carbohydrate) and sugar (simple carbohydrate) provide the body with energy. Fiber helps the intestine to get rid of waste products and can also help lower bad (LDL) cholesterol.

Simple Carbohydrate

The history of simple carbohydrate begins with sugar cane, which Christopher Columbus brought to the New World in the 1400s. Centuries later, sugar cane is cultivated in most countries and its products (table sugar and molasses) have become staple sources of food for the majority of the world. While simple carbohydrates can be found naturally, for example,

CHOOSING BETTER CARBOHYDRATES

Although low-carbohydrate or no-carbohydrate diets can help you lose weight in the short term, they are not sustainable in the long term and are not feasible as a lifelong practice. Your body needs carbohydrates to function. Just be smart about the carbohydrates you choose. Even though different foods may contain the same grams of sugar or starch, the foods you choose should also contain other nutrients and fewer additives.

Fiber-filled oatmeal might seem like a smart option for starting the day, but beware—there are levels of goodness for this popular breakfast choice. While oatmeal is full of fiber, watch out for hidden sugars in the prepackaged flavored varieties, which are very high in added—and unnecessary—sugar. Instead, opt for original plain oats jazzed up with fruit and flavors such as a dash of cinnamon or a drop of pure vanilla extract. The best choice is steel cut oats because the grain is intact and the fiber content high. It takes longer to cook, but it's worth it. We like to cook it with milk on the stovetop for a nice creamy texture.

Even though fruits and dairy products contain sugar naturally (lactose in dairy products is a type of sugar, and so is fructose in fruit), these foods are much better choices than juices, sodas, or muffins, which contain added sugar and preservatives to "enhance" the flavor. Remember that fruits also contain fiber and vitamins and minerals, and dairy products give you protein and calcium.

in fruit and dairy products, a typical Western diet contains added sugar in the form of processed foods such as candy, soda, cookies, and cakes. These high-sugar, high-calorie processed foods and beverages are contributing to the epidemic of obesity and obesity-related diseases such as diabetes, heart disease, and non-alcoholic fatty liver disease. While a whole fruit contains sugar, it also contains fiber and other nutrients that are beneficial and are a much better way to satisfy your sweet tooth and get the short-term energy you need.

Complex Carbohydrate

Complex carbohydrate, or starch, includes whole grains (such as rice, wheat, oats, and barley), root vegetables (such as potatoes, yams, and cassava), and legumes (such as beans, lentils, peanuts, and peas). Carbohydrates that contain fiber make you feel full and also help your intestines get rid of wastes and toxins. Good carbohydrates are minimally processed foods that are high in fiber and other nutrients, such as fruits, root vegetables, whole grains, legumes, and whole-grain bread and pasta. Bad carbohydrates are foods that are high in calories but low in fiber and other nutrients, such as sodas, candy, cakes, cookies, and white bread.

Fiber

Fiber is not digested by the body. Rather, it passes through the body and helps regulate blood sugar, keeps hunger at bay, and contributes to the health of many organs. There are two kinds of fiber, both essential to the body.

Soluble fiber helps lower blood glucose levels and blood cholesterol. Bile acids dissolve soluble fiber in the intestines to form a "gel" that is passed from the body in stools. Excellent sources of soluble fiber include oatmeal, nuts, beans, lentils, apples, oranges, flaxseeds, cucumber, celery, carrots, strawberries, pears, and blueberries.

Insoluble fiber does not dissolve in water but passes through the digestive tract adding bulk and softness to the stools. It promotes good bowel health and prevents constipation. Good sources of insoluble fiber include whole grains (such as brown rice, barley, and wheat bran), carrots, cucumbers, zucchini, cabbage, grapes, dark leafy vegetables, broccoli, green beans, tomatoes, and the skins of root vegetables.

Oat bran (the outer coating of oats) contains both soluble and insoluble fiber. Readily available in stores, it can be cooked the same way as oatmeal, with milk and fruit.

Protein

The second largest energy source after carbohydrate, protein is the building block of the human body. It is essential for tissue repair, proper functioning of the immune system, and hundreds of other vital duties.

The liver makes many of the essential proteins that are released into the bloodstream for use where the body needs them. Patients with liver injuries risk poor healing of tissues, delayed liver regeneration, and muscle wasting if they do not get adequate protein. The most common sources of protein are poultry, seafood, meat, dairy products, eggs, and plant sources such as beans and lentils.

It is important to eat both animal and plant proteins every day. If you are vegetarian, you can meet your protein needs with plant sources, but talk to your doctor about screening for iron and other nutrient deficiencies that may require you to take supplements.

Choose protein foods wisely. Opt for lean proteins such as chicken, fish, and beans instead of red meat. Steam, grill, bake, stir-fry, braise, or roast your lean protein with lots of herbs, spices, garlic, onions, and vegetables instead of deep-frying and heavily salting.

Fat

The largest store of energy in the body, fat has several functions, including insulation to regulate body temperature, protecting the organs by padding them, and aiding absorption of important vitamins. However, most Americans consume excess fat, which accumulates in the liver and damages it. Not all fat in food is the same. There is healthy fat, which is unsaturated, and unhealthy fat, consisting of saturated fat as well as trans fat, which harms the liver, heart, and kidneys. Keep in mind that fat has a high calorie content (9 calories per gram), so it's important not to eat too much, even if it is healthy fat.

Saturated fat. This fat comes mainly from animal sources such as red meat, poultry skin, and full-fat dairy products. It is better to choose lean cuts of meat and poultry without skin, and limit dairy products such as ice cream. However, in the case of malnourished patients with liver disease, it is acceptable to choose full-fat dairy products and fattier cuts of meat and poultry.

Trans fat. This fat is manufactured from oils using a method called partial hydrogenation. Research shows that trans fat increases unhealthy (LDL) cholesterol and decreases healthy (HDL) cholesterol.

The good unsaturated fat helps lower cholesterol, reduces the risk of heart disease, helps manage moods, keeps your brain alert, and fights fatigue. Remember, these foods contain high amount of calories, and moderation is the key! But eaten in the right amount, they may help with weight loss.

Monounsaturated fat (MUFA). This type of fat improves cholesterol and insulin levels, and helps control blood sugar. It is found in vegetable oils, seeds, nuts, and avocados.

Polyunsaturated fat (PUFA). Found mainly in plant-based foods, this fat is beneficial to the heart and decreases the risk of type 2 diabetes. It is found in vegetable oils, fish, and seafood.

Omega-3 fatty acids. A type of polyunsaturated fat, omega-3s are found in both plant and non-plant sources. However, the body is better able to convert omega-3s from fish than from plant sources. Fish high in omega-3s include salmon, tuna, mackerel, trout, sardines, and herring. Plant sources include olive, safflower, and peanut oils.

Omega-6 fatty acids. Also a type of polyunsaturated fat, omega-6s are found in seed oils such as canola, rapeseed, and cottonseed. Some of these oils are used to deep-fry foods, but you should stay away from deep-fried foods entirely, regardless of the oil used.

Cholesterol. Although cholesterol is not fat, you should be aware of its role in building cells and making certain hormones. The body makes enough cholesterol to meet its needs and does not require additional cholesterol from foods. Foods high in saturated fat are also high in cholesterol, so avoiding these foods will help decrease the intake of both saturated fat and cholesterol. Note that tropical oils such as coconut oil contain saturated fat but no cholesterol.

Overall, avoid deep-fried foods, processed foods, and baked goods containing saturated fat and trans fat. You will become knowledgeable as you start reading food labels and the ingredients lists on packaged food.

Micronutrients

The body needs small quantities of micronutrients such as vitamins and minerals to keep itself functioning well. The following are important micronutrients that anyone with liver disease—or who wants to avoid liver problems—should be aware of.

Water-Soluble Vitamins

These vitamins dissolve in water, so when the body absorbs what it needs, the excess passes from the body in urine.

Vitamin B1 (thiamine). Needed by the body for efficient carbohydrate use, vitamin B1 is found in meat, nuts, beans, and whole grains. It is crucial that patients with a history of alcohol abuse stop drinking and include a diet rich in this vitamin because they are at high risk of developing Wernicke's encephalopathy, which is caused by vitamin B1 deficiency. This condition can be treated but is fatal if not recognized in a timely manner and treated. The symptoms include confusion and loss of mental activity leading to coma and death. Other symptoms include loss of muscle coordination and vision changes.

Vitamin B3 (niacin/nicotinic acid). Vitamin B3 is also important in helping the body utilize carbohydrates efficiently. Patients with a history of heavy alcohol use and malnutrition are at high risk of developing vitamin B3 deficiency. This vitamin is readily available in fish, grains, dates, avocados, nuts, and mushrooms.

Vitamin B6 (pyridoxine). Among the crucial roles vitamin B6 plays are protecting the heart and making chemicals that transmit signals in the brain. B6 supplementation is widely used for various conditions to ease nerve pain, increase appetite, and relieve muscle cramps. People with severe liver disease are at risk of vitamin B6 deficiency because the liver is where B6 is processed. The vitamin is found in meats, whole grains, vegetables, nuts, bananas, avocados, and eggs.

Vitamin B9 (folate/folic acid). Folate is essential for cell growth and repair throughout the body. Folate deficiency can result in anemia, confusion, nerve damage, and greater liver injury from alcohol. A deficiency is common in patients with liver disease, especially heavy alcohol users, because alcohol interferes with absorption of the vitamin. Good sources of folate are spinach and other leafy green vegetables, broccoli, beans, peas, lentils, bananas, melons, and fortified whole-grain breads and cereals.

Vitamin B12 (cobalamin). B12 plays a major role in the normal functioning of the brain and nervous system, and in blood formation. It is found in animal sources such as fish, shellfish, poultry, eggs, milk, and milk products. If you are a vegetarian or vegan, you may need supplementation—but check with your doctor first. B12 is added to most multivitamins and is better absorbed when taken with other B vitamins.

Vitamin C (ascorbic acid). This vitamin offers many benefits such as protecting against cardiovascular disease, boosting the immune system, reducing the risk of eye diseases, and improving dental health. It also helps with iron absorption, wound healing, bone maintenance, repair and maintenance of cartilage, and collagen formation. Citrus fruits, tomatoes, papaya, mango, watermelon, cantaloupe, dark leafy greens, cauliflower, broccoli, brussels sprouts, and many vegetables are good sources of vitamin C.

Smoking tobacco inhibits absorption of vitamin C, and a poor diet can lead to a deficiency. Choose your sources of vitamin C wisely—it's always better to choose a whole orange with all its fiber rather than a glass of orange juice, which has excess sugar (since it is equivalent to eating more than 1 orange) and little or no fiber.

Choline. Choline is usually grouped with B-vitamins, and it is needed for all cells to maintain their integrity and is used as a neurotransmitter, required to transport fat molecules from the liver. Research shows that deficiency can cause fatty liver disease. Some of the major food sources of choline are eggs, legumes, and wheat germ, and it's easy to obtain enough choline by including these in your daily diet.

Fat-Soluble Vitamins

Patients with cholestatic liver diseases may be deficient in fat-soluble vitamins since they lack an adequate supply of bile salts to help the intestines absorb these vitamins. Fat-soluble vitamins are contained in fat globules, which are hard for the intestines to absorb. Bile acids break up the fat globules into little droplets so that the vitamins can be absorbed.

Vitamin A. Required for proper development and functioning of eyes, skin, and the immune system, vitamin A is found in carrots, eggs, fruits, whole milk, and butter. Vitamin A deficiency, common in patients with cholestatic liver diseases, may result in poor bone growth and increased risk of infection. Talk to your doctor about whether you need a supplement and, if you do, the right dose since too much vitamin A is toxic to the liver.

Vitamin D. This vitamin is important for the absorption of calcium, and for bone health and immune function. Patients with alcoholic liver disease are prone to vitamin D deficiency due to malabsorption caused by poor nutrition and possibly to inadequate sun exposure. While the sun is a good source of vitamin D, the risk of skin cancer limits it as a preferred source. Vitamin D is found in a natural state only in small quantities in certain foods; for example, fatty fish such as sardines, herring, mackerel, salmon, and tuna. Dairy products are often fortified with vitamin D—check the label. A simple blood test can determine whether you are deficient in vitamin D and need supplementation.

Vitamin E. Important for proper functioning of the brain and nervous system, vitamin E has been shown to help non-alcoholic fatty liver disease patients. This vitamin is considered an antioxidant and is found in many foods such as vegetable cooking oil, poultry, eggs, whole-grain cereals, wheat germ, spinach, kale, broccoli, collard greens, avocados, and nuts, especially almonds.

Vitamin K. Necessary for blood clotting, vitamin K is found in leafy green vegetables such as spinach and kale, and in broccoli, brussels sprouts, cabbage, and asparagus.

Essential Minerals

Let's talk about some minerals that are especially important for people with liver disease.

Calcium. Crucial in the formation and health of bones and teeth, calcium is also found in the blood and muscles. Milk and other dairy products, kale, and broccoli are among calcium-rich foods. People with any liver disease are encouraged to eat a diet rich in calcium and vitamin D. Avoid alcohol, which has been shown to be directly harmful to bone cells and may negatively affect calcium absorption. Tobacco use, lack of exercise, certain medications, and hormonal imbalance also contribute to bone loss. Calcium supplementation should be done carefully under medical supervision, because too much calcium leads to deficiencies of other essential micronutrients.

Iron. A key mineral, iron helps the body make hemoglobin and transports oxygen throughout the cells. Liver patients commonly have iron deficiency anemia, which results from blood loss through the gastrointestinal tract. The heme form of iron is found in animal sources such as red meat, poultry, and fish. The non-heme form is available in animal sources as well as plant sources such as spinach, dried fruits such as raisins and apricots, peas, and many fortified breads, cereals, and pasta. Heme iron is more easily absorbed by the body and can promote the absorption of non-heme iron. For example, eating beef with spinach helps your body absorb iron from the spinach. Vitamin C also promotes the absorption of both heme and non-heme iron, while calcium, phytic acid (found in the hulls of nuts, seeds, and grains), and tannic acid (found in black and pekoe teas, coffee, cola drinks, chocolate, and red wine) prevent the absorption of iron. So having an orange as dessert after having a meal with beef will increase iron absorption while drinking either milk or red wine with beef will decrease iron absorption.

People with hemochromatosis or another form of iron overload or cirrhosis should avoid any iron supplements or vitamins containing iron. If you have iron overload, talk to your doctor about whether you need to avoid certain foods.

Potassium. A diet high in potassium lowers blood pressure (thus decreasing the risk of stroke and heart disease), protects bones, and reduces the risk of kidney stones. Lower potassium levels are associated with increased risk of non-alcoholic fatty liver disease. People with liver disease have been found to have a low total body store of potassium. Potassium-rich foods include potatoes, tomatoes, avocados, fresh fruits (such as bananas, oranges, and strawberries), dried fruits (such as raisins, apricots, prunes, and dates), spinach, beans, and peas. Boiling strips the potassium content, so eat the fruits and vegetables raw when possible. Otherwise, roast or lightly steam them to preserve as much potassium as possible. If you are on diuretics (medications to make you urinate), your doctor will have to monitor your potassium level. Discuss with your doctor how much potassium you should be consuming.

Copper. This mineral helps the body make red blood cells and collagen, as well as keeps the nerves and immune system healthy. Copper is found in seafood, dried fruits, mushrooms, liver, chocolate, nuts, legumes, and wheat bran cereals. Although generally rare, copper deficiency is common in patients who have been receiving intravenous artificial feeding solutions. If copper deficiency is diagnosed, supplementation should be under medical supervision. A rare disorder called Wilson's disease causes copper buildup in the body (see page 24). Anyone with Wilson's disease should avoid foods high in copper.

Zinc. Needed on a daily basis because the body cannot store it, zinc plays a huge role in helping more than 100 enzymes perform their duties. Oysters are the major source of zinc, but red meat, poultry, whole grains, dairy products, and fortified breakfast cereals are the other most common sources. Chronic use of steroids, poor absorption in the gastrointestinal tract, and pancreatic insufficiency all can lead to zinc deficiency.

Zinc deficiency impairs a person's ability to smell and taste food. People with liver disease often complain that even their once-favorite foods are not tempting or do not taste the same. If you have these symptoms, talk to your doctor.

Healthy Portion Sizes

Portion sizes in the United States have grown dramatically over the past 20 years. In fact, the portions served in American restaurants have doubled and tripled over this period. For example, a typical bagel has more than doubled in size, and a blueberry muffin has more than tripled. This has led to what is called "portion distortion." Because of the inflated portion sizes, we have now come to think of restaurant portions as normal. Along with more added sugar and processed foods, the sharp increase in portion sizes has led to the epidemic of obesity and obesity-related diseases. As a country, we have been eating worse and eating too much. The first step in eating healthier is knowing what a healthy portion size is, learning how many servings of each food group are ideal, and finding out how to read food labels.

Let's start with some definitions. A "portion" is the amount of food that you choose to eat for a meal or a snack. A "serving" is a measured amount of food, such as 1 cup (8 ounces) of milk or one slice of bread. If you decide to have a sandwich with two slices of bread and one 8-ounce glass of milk, then you are having two servings of bread or carbohydrate, one serving of milk or dairy, and whatever you are putting into your sandwich. The serving sizes are determined by the USDA's MyPlate (United States Department of Agriculture) and the FDA (Food and Drug Administration).

We need to retrain our eyes and minds on what a normal portion is. While ideal portion sizes vary from person to person depending on factors including state of health, here are some easy tips to help you estimate portion sizes without have to tote around measuring cups. Depending on your specific condition and nutritional needs, your serving sizes will increase or decrease.

Recommended Serving Sizes

NUTRIENT	SERVING SIZE (CHOOSE ONE)	VISUAL EQUIVALENT	SERVINGS/DAY
Carbohydrates	½ cup cooked rice or pasta 1 slice bread ½ cup cooked cereal 1 cup ready-to-eat cereal 1 small sweet potato	1 cup is about a closed fist.	5
Protein	3–4 ounces of meat, poultry, or seafood ¼ cup cooked beans 1 egg 1 tablespoon peanut butter ½ ounce nuts or seeds	3–4 ounces of meat, poultry, or seafood is about the size of your palm. 1 tablespoon of peanut butter is about the size of a thumb.	3
Nuts and dried fruits	1 ounce	1 ounce is about a handful.	
Healthy fat (saturated fat should be less than 7% of total caloric intake for the day)	1 tablespoon peanut butter 1 teaspoon olive oil, canola oil, vegetable oil, or unsalted butter ⅛ of an average size avocado	1 tablespoon of peanut butter is about the size of a thumb.	3
Dairy	1 cup (8 ounces) milk or yogurt 2 cups cottage cheese 1½ ounces hard cheese	1 cup is about a closed fist. 1½ ounces hard cheese is about the size of a matchbox.	3
Fruits and vegetables	1 cup fruit 1 cup cooked or raw vegetables 2 cups raw leafy greens	1 cup is about a closed fist.	6–7
Sodium	No more than 2,300 mg/day, ideally around 1,500 mg/day		Less than 2,300 mg
Processed sugar	Less than 6 teaspoons for women Less than 9 teaspoons for men		Less than 6 teaspoons (22 grams) for women, less than 9 teaspoons (33 grams) for men
Fiber			20 grams for women, 30 grams for men

Reading Food Labels

There is so much information on the nutrition labels of packaged foods that some of it is helpful and some of it is confusing. When reading a label, pay attention to the "Nutrition Facts" panel. At the top of the panel is the serving size and the number of servings per container, followed by the number of calories and the total fat grams per serving broken down by fat type. Next come the amounts of sodium, sugar, fiber, and protein.

When you keep track of what you eat (for example, the amount of sodium, calories, and sugar), be sure to multiply by the number of servings you consume. For example, the nutrition facts panel on a pint tub of ice cream may tell you that a serving size is ½ cup, there are 4 servings in the container, and each serving is 270 calories. If you eat half of the pint, you are eating 2 servings. So the amount of calories you consumed is 540 (270 calories per serving × 2).

Nutrition Facts

Serving Size 1 cup (228g)
Servings per Container 2

Amount per Serving

Calories 250	Calories from Fat 110

	% Daily Value*
Total Fat 12g	18%
Saturated Fat 3g	15%
Trans Fat 1.5g	
Cholesterol 30mg	10%
Sodium 470mg	20%
Total Carbohydrate 31g	10%
Dietary Fiber 0g	0%
Sugars 5g	
Protein 5g	

Vitamin A 4%	•	Calcium 20%
Vitamin C 2%	•	Iron 4%

* Percent Daily Values are based on a 2,000 calorie diet. Your Daily Values may be higher or lower depending on your calorie needs:

	Calories:	2,000	2,500
Total Fat	Less than	65g	80g
Sat Fat	Less than	20g	25g
Cholesterol	Less than	300mg	300mg
Sodium	Less than	2,400mg	2,400mg
Total Carbohydrate		300g	375g
Dietary Fiber		25g	30g

You will want to look for foods that do not contain trans fat; are low in saturated fat, sodium, and sugar; and are high in fiber and protein. To figure out how much fat, sodium, sugar, fiber, or protein the food contains, you must multiply the amount on the label by the number of servings you are having. This is especially important in keeping accurate count of your sodium intake. For example, a typical can of soup contains 2 servings. If the nutrition facts panel states that there are 1,000 mg of sodium per serving, then you are taking in 2,000 mg of sodium if you have the whole can of soup (1,000 mg × 2 servings).

The relatively new "front of package labeling" lists the number of calories and the amounts of saturated fat, sodium, sugar, and fiber right on the front of the container in an easy-to-read format.

Finally, take heed of the ingredients list, which itemizes the ingredients in descending order by weight. This means that the item contains the most of the first ingredient by weight, and the least of the last ingredient by weight. Note that some foods that we think of as healthy, such as oatmeal and yogurt, can come with a large amount of added sugar. Plain yogurt and milk have naturally occurring sugar, which show up on the nutrition facts panel. However, you should not see sugar as one of the listed ingredients in plain yogurt and milk. There are sweetened, flavored yogurts and oatmeal with added sugar. These will list sugar or other sweeteners in the ingredients list, often as the second ingredient—meaning that after milk or oatmeal, the largest component of what you are eating is added sugar. That's why reading the ingredients list is very important.

Watch out for the following terms on an ingredients list. Each one means that sugar has been added to the product.

- High fructose corn syrup

- Corn sweetener

- Corn syrup

- Evaporated cane juice

- Fruit juice concentrates

- Malt sugar

- Sugar names ending in "-ose" (dextrose, fructose, maltose, sucrose)

- Syrup

Note: Currently, the Food and Drug Administration is proposing changes to the decades-old nutrition facts panel. While the final version is still pending, the proposed changes aim to have serving size more closely reflect correct portion size. The proposed changes also include adding more information on sugar, and listing vitamin D and potassium content.

When reading labels, do not be swayed by claims such as "all natural," "low fat," "low sodium," "lower sugar," or "organic." Read the nutrition facts panel and the ingredients list, and judge for yourself whether that product fits a healthy lifestyle. "All natural" does not necessarily mean that the product does not contain added sugar, sodium, or saturated fats. "Low fat" does not necessarily mean that all the fat is healthy fat. "Low sodium" may simply mean that the product contains less sodium than the typical equivalent product, but it may still have more sodium than you want. For example, a canned soup that claims to be low in sodium may have 750 mg of sodium instead of 1,000 mg. One can (2 servings) of this "low-sodium soup" will give you 1,500 mg of sodium—what you should consume for almost the whole day!

Also, don't be fooled by the word "organic," which implies healthy but sometimes isn't. Although the USDA certified organic label means that at least 70% of the ingredients are certified organic (not grown or produced with synthetic chemicals, irradiation, or sewage sludge), it can still contain too much sugar, sodium, or saturated fat. For example, USDA certified organic sodas are still sodas that contain added sugar without other beneficial nutrients.

CHAPTER 4

DETOXIFY YOUR BODY

Over the years, the standard American diet has adopted an abundance of highly processed foods. A hectic and fast-paced lifestyle means Americans spend less time in the kitchen cooking wholesome, real food and more time eating on the go. We look to packaged products for quick meals. This foodstuff is packed with added sodium, sugar, and unhealthy fat. We eat out at fast food restaurants, where the food is laden with saturated fat and sodium. Fast food is void of nutrients and, more important, responsible for a diet that is toxic to our bodies. This toxic diet is one of the leading causes of the most common liver disease in the United States, non-alcoholic fatty liver disease—which, fortunately, is reversible with a healthy diet. We need to get back to the basics of what the liver is meant to process, and it's not fast food or processed food. For the liver to function properly and rid the body of toxins, we must cut out those unhealthy foods, increase hydration, increase fiber, and get moving.

Eliminate Toxins

The first step in detoxing is to eliminate or reduce the things that are toxic to you. These can be foods, drinks, or even household products that you use on a daily basis.

Eliminate Added Sugar

Your liver has to process and store the sugar that you eat. Excess sugar intake can make your liver fatty and inflamed, resulting in liver damage. Added sugar is high in calories, leading to weight gain, which further damages the liver.

There are several different ways to eliminate added sugar, including avoiding sugary beverages, baked goods, and processed foods commonly made with a lot of added sugar. First and foremost, read the ingredients lists on the foods in your pantry and refrigerator. You might be surprised by the items containing large amounts of sugar, such as tomato sauce. Clear your pantry and refrigerator of foods with added sugar, including:

- Sodas, juices, sweetened iced tea, sports drinks, and any other sweetened drinks (including chocolate milk).

- Sweetened cold and hot cereals such as Cocoa Puffs, Froot Loops and other cereals with "fruit flavors," and flavored-sweetened oatmeal. Some cereals are marketed to look healthy (advertising that they are fortified with vitamins and minerals), but most are full of sugar.

- Cookies, pastries, cakes, and other sweets.

- Sweetened, flavored yogurt.

- Processed foods in general.

Here are other ways to cut down on sugar:

Reduce sweetness in your coffee or tea. Gradually add less and less sugar or honey until you don't crave that sweetness any more.

Eat fruit. Get your sugar from natural sources like fruit, which is full of fiber. Your body utilizes the fiber in the process of digestion, making the sugar in fruit break down more slowly. The end result is that you stay full longer than if you had eaten refined sugar.

Limit dessert. If you are used to eating dessert after lunch and dinner, reduce it to once a day and then to a few times a week until your cravings subside.

Portion your sugar. If you do need a nibble of chocolate here and there, we get it. It's fine as long as it is just a nibble. Take a square or two of chocolate and then put the bar away so that you will not be tempted to eat more.

Use sugar substitutes. Apple sauce, molasses, and palm sugar (which is extracted from the sap of palm trees) are wonderful substitutes for refined white sugar when you're baking cookies or cakes.

Eliminate High-Sodium Foods

Patients with cirrhosis are prone to accumulating fluid in the belly and throughout the body. Lower your sodium intake by not adding salt to foods and by not eating out.

Most people think that salt is the just the table salt added to foods. However, it is a natural component of many foods and has been added liberally to most processed foods. It goes by many names, including monosodium glutamate, sea salt, disodium phosphate, baking soda, and sodium citrate. The reason it is found in almost all processed foods is because it is added as a flavor enhancer, seasoning agent, and preservative.

Avoid using salt when cooking. Table salt, sea salt, kosher salt—they are all salt! Gradually cut back on the amount of salt you put in or on your food.

Use herbs and spices. Most of us have learned to use salt as the fallback for flavoring food. There are so many more exciting ways to spice up your food than with salt. To help you eliminate sodium from your diet, here are some herbs and spices that you can use:

LEAN RED MEATS	Coriander, cumin, horseradish, mustard, oregano, paprika, rosemary, and thyme.
FISH AND SEAFOOD	Citrus, cumin, dill, garlic, ginger, oregano, paprika, saffron, tarragon, thyme, and turmeric.
POULTRY	Citrus, coriander, cumin, curry, dill, garlic, ginger, rosemary, saffron, sage, tarragon, and turmeric.
EGGS	Basil, chili powder, cilantro, cumin, curry, dill, paprika, tarragon, and thyme.
BEANS	Basil, chili powder, cloves, coriander, cumin, oregano, rosemary, and turmeric.
FRUITS	Cardamom, cinnamon, cloves, ginger, and nutmeg.
VEGETABLES	Basil, citrus, cumin, ginger, paprika, and tarragon.

Leave the salt shaker off the table. If it's not sitting right in front of you, you'll think twice before using it.

Eliminate canned and jarred foods. Salt is used as a preservative in canned and jarred vegetables, sauces, soups, beans, sauces, and other foods. Preservatives are added to keep the contents "fresh." How can food be nutritious if its shelf life is 2 to 3 years?

Stop using condiments. Condiments such as pickles, soy sauce, pasta sauce, barbecue sauce, ready-to-cook sauces (such as Indian, Mexican, and Thai), and dips all contain a lot of sodium.

Cut out packaged foods. Yes, that means chips, crackers, microwave popcorn, and other snack items.

Stop eating frozen meals. Frozen, processed, ready-to-eat meals are laden with salt, just as canned and jarred products are.

Stop eating deli meats. Cold cuts, sausages, bacon, and other cured meats contain a lot of sodium.

Reduce Saturated Fat

Eating a diet high in saturated fat has been shown to increase visceral fat and fat deposits in the liver (non-alcoholic fatty liver disease). Visceral fat—abdominal fat that is wrapped around organs—increases the risk of diabetes, heart disease, stroke, and even dementia. You do not have to be

UNDERSTANDING POPULAR DIETS

If you are carrying excess weight, by now you know you need to lose it to benefit your liver health as well as your overall well-being. You have probably come across fad diets. Perhaps a friend or family member is on one, or maybe you learned about such a diet on TV, in a magazine, or online. Fad diets are quick ways to help you lose weight, but we do not recommend them. We generally advise our patients against diets that cut out entire food groups, last for a limited time period, or rely on prepared meals.

Diets that cut out entire food groups such as grains, legumes, and dairy put you at risk for nutrient deficiencies. These diets are not sustainable. It takes an immense amount of self-control to give up entire food groups that you are accustomed to eating regularly. This leads to the yo-yo effect, where your weight fluctuates back and forth. When you are on the diet, you shed pounds—but as soon as you go back to old habits, you gain even more weight. The yo-yo-ing can decrease your metabolism and make it even harder to lose weight.

As for prepared meals, they are expensive and most people do not want to eat them on a permanent basis. The problem we find with plans that sell prepared meals is that once people stop buying the food, they are back on their own and have not learned how to prepare healthy meals. They revert to old habits and regain the weight.

We do not recommend the paleo diet, the South Beach diet, the zone diet, the Atkins diet, the raw food diet, Nutrisystem, or the macrobiotic diet. The two diets that we feel are healthy for someone with liver disease are the DASH diet and the Mediterranean diet.

DASH Diet

DASH (Dietary Approaches to Stop Hypertension) is especially recommended for people with high or borderline high blood pressure. Left untreated, hypertension increases the risk of heart disease, stroke, kidney disease, and blindness. The DASH diet is proven to lower blood pressure in about 2 weeks and is endorsed by organizations such as the National Heart, Lung and Blood Institute; the American Heart Association; the

2010 Dietary Guidelines for Americans; the U.S. guidelines for treatment of high blood pressure; and Mayo Clinic.

The core of the DASH diet is eating a diet rich in fruits, vegetables, whole grains, and low-fat dairy while limiting added sugar, added fat, and red meat. The diet is thought to lower blood pressure because food choices are low in sodium and high in potassium, calcium, and magnesium.

There are two versions of the diet. The standard DASH diet allows 2,300 mg of sodium per day (equivalent to 1 teaspoon of salt). The lower sodium DASH diet, allowing up to 1,500 mg of sodium per day, is usually recommended for people who are 51 or older, are black, or have hypertension, diabetes, or chronic kidney disease.

FOODS ALLOWED:

Vegetables: 4 to 5 servings per day

Fruits: 4 to 5 servings per day

Low-fat dairy foods: 2 to 3 servings per day

Whole grains: 6 to 8 servings per day

Lean meat, fish, and poultry: 6 or fewer servings per day

Fats and oils: 2 to 3 servings per day

Nuts, seeds, and legumes: 4 to 5 servings per week

Sweets: 5 or fewer servings per week

The DASH diet is a healthy way to eat. In addition to lowering blood pressure, its many health benefits include helping to prevent osteoporosis, cancer, heart disease, stroke, and diabetes. The diet is consistent with our low-sodium recommendations for liver patients, and it offers similar serving sizes of whole grains, lean proteins, and fruits and vegetables that we recommend on page 44.

Mediterranean Diet

This diet is a heart-healthy eating plan modeled on the basic nutritious regimen that people in Mediterranean countries have followed for centuries. The diet consists of mostly plant-based foods like whole grains, legumes, fruits, and vegetables. Fish and other lean protein, and low-fat dairy are also key elements. Olive oil is the main source of fat. Extra virgin and virgin are the least processed forms of olive oil containing the highest levels of protective compounds for maximum health benefits.

The Mediterranean diet is not about counting calories or servings per day. It is about changing the foods you put into your body, and limiting saturated fat and refined carbohydrates. Greeks are known to consume six or more antioxidant-rich fruits and vegetables per day. Throughout the Mediterranean region, bread is either eaten plain or dipped in olive oil rather than being slathered with butter or margarine.

The main principles are:

- Eating mostly plant-based foods—whole grains, legumes, fruits, vegetables, and nuts—every day. (Limit nuts to a handful per day.)

- Replacing butter with olive oil/canola.

- Using herbs and spices instead of salt to flavor foods.

- Choosing low-fat dairy products.

- Limiting red meat to a few times a month.

- Eating fish and poultry at least twice a week.

- Drinking red wine in moderation (optional).

- Engaging in physical activity.

This is a lifestyle change that can have lasting positive effects, such as good heart and mental health as proved by clinical research. This diet is also consistent with the recommendations for healthier fat and high fiber that we give to our liver patients.

obese to have visceral fat, so even if you are slender, you should cut down on saturated fat.

USDA recommends that healthy adults over 19 get between 20% to 35% of their daily calories from fat and less than 7% of saturated fat in a day. However, in people with liver disease or other medical conditions, this percentage varies. Consult a registered dietitian for a recommendation specific to your situation. Here are some ways to cut saturated fat and trans fat from your diet, and to incorporate healthy fat.

Eliminate processed foods. See a pattern? These foods tend to be high in saturated fat as well as sodium and sugar.

Limit red meat to one or two times per week. Chances are you won't miss having so much red meat but instead will look forward to the one or two meals when you do have it.

Use ground turkey instead of ground beef. For hamburgers, tacos, and stir-fries, replace beef with lean turkey.

Stay away from cured meats. Not only are cured meats from the deli loaded with sodium, but they contain a lot of saturated fat.

Eliminate Herbal Supplements

Because the liver processes many prescription medications, over-the-counter medications, and herbal supplements, check with your doctor to be sure anything you plan to take is safe for your liver. Acetaminophen (Tylenol) can be taken safely at the right doses even if you have chronic liver disease. However, it is very important to limit acetaminophen to 2,000 mg a day. Acetaminophen is found in most over-the-counter cold and flu medicines, so make sure to account for all the doses you are taking. Taking too much can cause liver injury, or even liver failure.

Be aware that herbal supplements are not regulated by the Food and Drug Administration. Their efficacy and safety often are not well studied. There is a misconception that they give health benefits without any potential for harm. Like any foreign substance you put in your body, supplements have a potential for toxicity and for interactions with other medications. A 2010 congressional investigation found that herbal supplements were often contaminated with heavy metals and pesticides.

Eliminate Alcohol

The products that alcohol breaks down into can be toxic to your liver. Drinking too much alcohol can harm the liver by causing fat deposits, inflammation, and cirrhosis. If you have a chronic liver disease, such as hepatitis C, avoid alcohol altogether, because the combination of alcohol and hepatitis C causes even more severe damage. Alcohol can also make acetaminophen more toxic to your liver, and it can interact with a number of other medications. Because women produce less alcohol dehydrogenase, the enzyme that breaks down alcohol, they are more susceptible to the toxic effects of alcohol at lower amounts than men. And if you drink only wine or beer instead of liquor, that does not mean the wine or beer won't do the same amount of damage. Whether you drink a 12-ounce can or bottle of beer, a 5-ounce glass of wine, or 1½ ounces of distilled liquor, you're getting the same 14 grams of alcohol.

Eliminate Environmental Toxins

Chemical and heavy metals that you may come into contact with at work or home or in food may be toxic to your liver. To minimize these external exposures, follow these tips:

Use a good water filter. It will remove heavy metals from your drinking water.

Dispose of old cleaning agents, solvents, paint, and other chemicals. Very old chemicals may still contain banned toxins and heavy metals. Check with your local environmental or waste management agency on how to safely dispose of these chemicals. Do NOT throw them into the regular trash.

Avoid skin contact with cleaning, paint, or other chemical-containing products. Make sure your house is well ventilated during use of any chemicals.

Avoid using a thermometer that contains mercury. You'll find safer alternatives at your local drugstore or pharmacy.

Choose non-toxic household cleaners. Toxic organic content increases with the number and amount of additives. Choose plain products with fewer ingredients that don't contain chlorine, alcohol, triclosan, triclocarban, lye, glycol ether, or ammonia. Look for ones that are phosphate-free, VOC-free, and solvent-free. You can also try using some inexpensive homemade alternatives such as baking soda, unscented soaps, lemon, sodium borate (borax), vinegar, isopropyl alcohol, and cornstarch. Be sure to rinse surfaces thoroughly with water after using any household cleaner.

Check your house for lead or mercury paints. If you have a very old home, talk to a professional about having it checked for paint containing lead or mercury and other possible toxins.

The following are a few common chemicals that are especially detrimental to the liver.

Carbon Tetrachloride

Previously used in pesticides, refrigerant, dry cleaning solvent, cleaning products, and lava lamps, carbon tetrachloride was found to cause severe liver damage and liver failure. The production of it for use in consumer products was banned in the United States in 1970, but it is currently used in chemistry laboratories and in scientific research to understand liver injury. Although production was banned, common cleaning products may contain carbon tetrachloride as a result of chemical reactions from other ingredients in the cleaning products.

PCBs

Polychlorinated biphenyls, or PCBs, were once widely used in many products such as coolants, electrical wiring, electronic components, pesticides, cutting oil, flame retardant, lubricating oil, hydraulic fluids, sealants, adhesives, wood floor finishes, paints, waterproofing compounds, vacuum pump fluids, surgical implants, and fixatives. The production of

PCBs was banned in the United States in 1979 because of its known toxic effects. However, there have been high levels of PCBs found in wastewater sludge, soil, rivers, and lakes, and the consumption of fish from certain bodies of water has been restricted or banned. Drinking water in the United States is tested to make sure that there is no PCB contamination.

Vinyl Chloride

In the past, vinyl chloride was used as an aerosol spray repellent and a refrigerant. Known to cause liver injury and a rare type of liver cancer, it is a common contaminant found near landfills and released by industries. Once released, it can enter the air and drinking water.

Heavy Metals

Heavy metals such as lead and mercury can also cause liver injury. Lead-based paint was banned in the United States in 1978. If you live in a house or condominium built before 1978 and have young children at home, make sure to get your house tested for lead. Mercury was used in old indoor latex paint (banned in 1990) and is found in mercury-containing thermometers and living organisms.

It can build up in organisms such as fish so that as you go up the food chain, the concentration of mercury increases. As big fish such as swordfish, shark, and king mackerel eat a lot of little fish, the amount of mercury in the big fish builds up. The Food and Drug Administration and the Environmental Protection Agency advise women of child-bearing age, nursing mothers, and young children to avoid swordfish, shark, king mackerel, and tilefish from the Gulf of Mexico, and to limit consumption of albacore tuna to less than 6 ounces per week, less than three 6-ounce servings per month, and consumption of all other fish and shellfish to no more than 12 ounces per week. However, keep in mind that the omega-3 fatty acids in fish help protect the heart and liver, and are important for neurological development in children. In general, choose smaller fish that are lower on the food chain to get the benefit of omega-3s while avoiding too much mercury. See the table of mercury levels in seafood below.

Mercury Levels in Seafood

HIGH (avoid)	HIGHER (limit to less than 18 ounces per month)	LOWER (limit to less than 36 ounces per month)	LOWEST (limit to less than 12 ounces per week)
Marlin	Chilean sea bass	Striped or black bass	Anchovies
Orange roughy	Bluefish	Carp	Butterfish
Tilefish	Grouper	Alaskan cod	Catfish
Swordfish	Mackerel	White Pacific croaker	Clam
Shark	Tuna (white albacore, yellowfin)	Pacific and Atlantic halibut	Crab (domestic)
King mackerel		Silverside/Jacksmelt	Crawfish/crayfish
Tuna (bigeye, ahi)		Lobster	Flounder
		Mahi mahi	Haddock
		Monkfish	Hake
		Perch (freshwater)	Herring
		Sablefish	Mackerel (North Atlantic, chub)
		Skate	Mullet
		Snapper	Oysters
		Sea trout (weakfish)	Perch (ocean)
		Tuna (chunk light canned, skipjack)	Plaice
			Salmon (canned, fresh)
			Sardines
			Scallops
			Shad (American)
			Shrimp
			Sole
			Squid
			Tilapia
			Trout (freshwater)
			Whitefish
			Whiting

Aflatoxin

Aflatoxin is a toxic and carcinogenic (cancer-causing) substance produced by certain types of fungi. Found in contaminated foods, aflatoxin can increase the risk of liver cancer more in patients with chronic hepatitis B infection than in anyone else. Foods commonly contaminated with aflatoxin are corn, soybeans, peanuts, and corn, soy, and peanut products from developing countries.

Take care to avoid foods that may be contaminated with aflatoxin.

Hydration—Flush Out the Toxins

Your body needs lots of water to flush out toxins. Water also makes you feel full. It is free and one of the best beverages around as it has zero calories and is usually easy to find. It helps replace fluids lost while the body is busy breathing, sweating, and removing waste products every minute of the day. Below are some tips to help you get on track with healthy hydration.

Invest in a reusable water bottle. It will save you money and help the environment. Carry it with you at all times.

Keep track of your daily water intake. Use the worksheet on page 154 to see if you are reaching the goal of at least eight 8-ounce servings of water per day.

Drink milk as a snack. Choose milk in between meals as a snack or a post-exercise recovery drink—whole milk if you need to increase calories, or nonfat or low-fat milk otherwise.

Infuse it. Try adding fresh-cut fruit such as slices of watermelon, berries, cucumber, lime, or lemon. There is nothing more refreshing or healthier than a nice cold glass of water infused with fruit. Invest in a water filter and pitcher, and let the slices of fruit soak in the chilled water.

Just order water. If you are dining at a restaurant or in your own home, choose water over beverages high in sugar such as sodas, juices, sweetened iced tea, or other sweetened drinks. Remember, having to process the sugar puts a strain on your liver. Put money you would have otherwise spent on these beverages into a jar toward a vacation or something to treat yourself.

Make water exciting! For a treat, add an occasional tiny splash of 100% natural juice to sparkling water. We particularly like 100% pomegranate juice, and just a couple of ounces in a large glass of water is sufficient.

Wake up and drink a glass of water. It's as simple as that. Drink 8 ounces of water right after you open your eyes in the morning. It will help wake you up, and it's a quick count toward your eight glasses a day.

CHAPTER 5

HEALTHY FOODS FOR A HEALTHY LIVER

Now that you've rid your home and kitchen of highly processed foods, replace them with foods high in fiber, protein, nutrients, and flavor. Add healthy fat now that you have eliminated unhealthy fat. Eat more fiber, which fills you up and helps you eliminate toxins from your body, and get some quality protein and nutrients to help your liver repair itself. Well-timed healthy snacks between meals will prevent you from overeating, get you burning calories more efficiently, and make you feel more energetic.

The best way to eat right is to cook right. In Part 3 of this book, we have provided a wide range of recipes so you can experiment with new foods and flavors. Stock your kitchen with the healthy staples you'll need for meal preparation. (See page 143 for a list of healthy essentials for your pantry, refrigerator, and freezer.) For now, let's get familiar with the foods that will help heal your liver.

Protein

Protein is an important energy source. It is also a building block of tissues in the body, and is vital for growth and repair. You need adequate protein in your diet to help your liver heal and regenerate. The liver creates different essential by-products from plant proteins than it does from animal proteins, so it is important to get a combination of the two in your diet. Eating both types of protein ensures that the liver receives various nutrients that help it heal while it performs its duties in the body.

Plant Proteins

These are protein-rich foods derived from plants, which contain protein but also fiber and other important and essential micronutrients and lower saturated fat than animal-based protein foods.

Nuts and nut butters. Nuts such as almonds, walnuts, cashews, and pecans are a good source of protein, essential fatty acids (which help the liver with repair and regeneration of some of its cells), vitamin E, folate, zinc, selenium, phosphorus, magnesium, iron, calcium, and choline. They are also a good source of fiber. Unsalted nut butters are a great way to add nuts to your diet as well.

Seeds. Sunflower, pumpkin, and other seeds contain omega-3 and omega-6 fatty acids, healthy fat, vitamin A, fiber, vitamin K, folate, iron, potassium, phosphorus, magnesium, selenium, and zinc.

Tofu. Rich in protein, tofu is also a source of monounsaturated fat, folate, calcium, magnesium, phosphorus, potassium, and selenium.

Legumes. Soy beans, kidney beans, chickpeas, and other beans and lentils are excellent sources of protein, omega-3 and omega-6 fatty acids, vitamin A, vitamin C, folate, calcium, iron, magnesium, potassium, phosphorus, magnesium, zinc, and selenium.

Animal Proteins

These are protein foods derived from animals. They are rich in nutrients but could also have high amounts of saturated fat, so you need to choose with caution.

Eggs. Eggs are rich in protein, monounsaturated fats, essential fatty acids, vitamin A, choline, calcium, magnesium, phosphorus, potassium, selenium, and fluoride.

Poultry. Chicken, turkey, and other lean poultry (without the skin) are good sources of protein, essential fatty acids, healthy fats, vitamin A, niacin, folate, pantothenic acid, zinc, and selenium.

Beef. Choose lean cuts of beef such as sirloin tip side steak, top or bottom round and roast steak, top sirloin steak, and eye of round roast or steak over fattier cuts like filet mignon, flap steak, skirt steak, porter house steak, T-bone steak, New York strip steak, and rib eye steak. (Check with your grocer or butcher if you are not sure about a cut, and check with the chef to make sure you get a lean cut when dining out). An easy tip to go by is that

PUMP UP THE PROTEIN IN YOUR DIET

Here are some healthy ways to make sure you are getting sufficient protein in your diet.

Choose smarter snacks. Instead of snacking on chips, candy bars, and donuts, opt for high-protein snacks that will keep you full longer and give your liver the building blocks it needs to repair itself. For example, make your own bean salad with whole wheat pita chips (page 111). Go for an apple with unsalted nut butter. Have nonfat or low-fat dairy such as plain yogurt with fruit. Snack on a handful of almonds or homemade trail mix.

Think of eggs at snack time. Munch on a hard-boiled egg anytime during the day.

Switch to Greek yogurt. Substitute Greek yogurt for sour cream and mayonnaise in recipes. It increases protein value and contains good bacteria.

Include protein in every meal. Incorporate a good protein source— such as lean meat, fish, poultry, or tofu—into each meal.

Eat eggs for breakfast. Instead of grabbing a muffin or donut, make yourself a healthy omelet (page 103).

Recover with milk. Choose a tall glass of nonfat milk for your post-workout recovery drink.

Don't forget grains. Cook with grains that contain protein, such as quinoa and Kamut.

if there is a "round," "chuck," or "loin" in the name, then it's a lean or extra-lean cut. Leaner cuts of beef also contain iron, vitamin K, folate, vitamin B12, magnesium, selenium, fluoride, and zinc.

Oily fish. Oily fish such as salmon, mackerel, tuna, trout, sardines, and herring contain good amounts of omega-3 fatty acids, healthy fat, vitamin A, niacin, folate, vitamin B12, calcium, magnesium, selenium, potassium, and phosphorus.

Dairy. Plain yogurt, Greek yogurt, milk, and certain naturally lower sodium cheeses (such as Swiss, Gruyère, ricotta, and nonfat cottage cheese) are excellent sources of protein, calcium, vitamin A, vitamin D, potassium, phosphorus, magnesium, choline, and folate.

Yogurt is a natural and cost-efficient way to get probiotics, good bacteria that help maintain balance in the gut. These good bacteria live in the digestive tract and help move food along. When people with liver disease take several medications, especially antibiotics, many of those good bacteria are lost. It's very important to replenish them.

Carbohydrates

Consuming the right carbs every day is vital for anyone, but especially for patients with non-alcoholic fatty liver disease (NAFLD) and non-alcoholic steatohepatitis (NASH), who must lose excess weight. A diet rich in healthy carbohydrates provides the body with fiber, which is filling and curbs hunger. Fiber also helps inhibit the absorption of fat and sugar, which can put a strain on the liver, and is food for the good bacteria in the gut. These bacteria help remove toxins from the body that must otherwise be processed by the liver. If that weren't enough, carbs provide vitamins and minerals that are essential for regulating organ systems and helping them function well.

Fruits and Vegetables

Eat your greens and a variety of other vegetables as well as fruits. They provide various nutrients that help the liver flush out toxins and function better. These foods are also rich in fiber, which acts like a sponge in your gut and cleans up unhealthy substances such as excess cholesterol and saturated fat. Both the surplus cholesterol and saturated fat impose a huge burden on the liver and heart. Fresh fruits and vegetables are ideal, but if fresh isn't available, opt for unsalted frozen produce. Avoid canned vegetables, which are high in sodium and contain preservatives, and canned fruits, which are loaded with sugar from added juice and preservatives.

Fruits

Apple. A relatively inexpensive, easy-to-find, widely available fruit, the apple helps correct common micronutrient deficiencies that most liver patients suffer from because of poor diet and malabsorption. Apples contain vitamins A and C, potassium, and some calcium.

Banana. Easily available just about anywhere throughout the year, bananas are inexpensive and loaded with nutrients including essential fatty acids, vitamin A, vitamin C, folate, niacin, choline, magnesium, potassium, phosphorus, and selenium.

Berries. Available fresh in summer, berries are sold year-round in the frozen food aisle. They are rich in essential fatty acids and vitamins A, C, and K, as well as choline, folate, calcium, magnesium, potassium, and phosphorus.

Dates. Not as regularly consumed in the standard American diet as other fruits, dates are easy to incorporate because of their natural sweetness. They are rich in vitamin A, choline, folate, calcium, magnesium, potassium, and phosphorus, which together can correct several deficiencies common in patients with hepatitis C or alcohol-induced liver disease.

Grapes. Widely available, grapes are rich in vitamins A, C, and K in addition to folate, magnesium, potassium, and phosphorus. The red varieties are rich in antioxidants, which help the liver to regenerate.

Mango, pineapple, and papaya. These exotic fruits are rich in essential fatty acids and vitamins A, C, E, and K, as well as folate, choline, potassium, and phosphorus.

Pear. The pear varieties most commonly found in the United States are Bartlett, d'Anjou, Bosc, Seckel, and Asian. One variety or another is available in supermarkets throughout the year. Pears contain omega-6 fatty acids, vitamin C, vitamin K, folate, choline, phosphorus, and potassium.

Pomegranate. This fruit, which has become popular in recent years, contains good amounts of omega-6 fatty acids and vitamins C, K, and E, in addition to folate, choline, magnesium, calcium, potassium, and phosphorus.

Watermelon and cantaloupe. Melons contain omega-6 fatty acids, vitamins A and C, and choline.

Citrus. The many types of citrus—oranges, lemons, limes, grapefruit, and more—are rich in essential fatty acids, vitamins A and C, choline, calcium, potassium, and phosphorus.

Vegetables

Avocados. A wonderful source of healthy fats, avocados also contain high amounts of folate, which is beneficial for anyone suffering from folate deficiency due to alcohol-induced liver dysfunction. Additionally, avocados contain vitamins A, C, E, and K, as well as niacin, pantothenic acid, choline, calcium, magnesium, potassium, and zinc.

Beets. The rich color is a clue that beets contain many important nutrients such as essential fatty acids, vitamins A and C, folate, choline, calcium, potassium, and phosphorus, but are also rich in betaine, an amino acid that helps the liver cleanse itself to a degree. Avoid canned beets, which are high in sodium and preservatives. Fresh beets are very easy to peel, and boiling or steaming will retain the nutrients.

Broccoli. Both the florets and stems contain essential fatty acids, vitamins A and C, folate, calcium, magnesium, phosphorus, potassium, and selenium. This combination of nutrients helps the liver recover from the damage caused by non-alcoholic fatty liver disease, alcohol-induced liver disease, and viral diseases.

Brussels sprouts. This underconsumed but highly nutritious member of the cabbage family has good amounts of vitamins A, C, K, as well as folate, and choline. It contains small amounts of calcium, potassium, and phosphorus.

Carrots. The common carrot is a good source of vitamin A, which is stored in the liver. It also contains trace amounts of vitamin K and potassium.

Cauliflower. Although often underrecognized as a nutritious vegetable, cauliflower is an easy way to provide your liver with essential fatty acids, vitamins A and C, folate, manganese, and phosphorus. Cauliflower helps protect healthy cells in the body.

Collard greens. This leafy vegetable contains essential fatty acids and vitamins A, C, E, and K, as well as folate, choline, calcium, potassium, and magnesium. The combination of micronutrients helps bind the bile in the digestive tract to excrete easily from the body.

Cucumber. An easy vegetable to incorporate into your diet, cucumbers are inexpensive and available throughout the year. They are mostly water but also contain vitamins A and K, choline, and small amounts of potassium. Cucumbers are a very hydrating vegetable that helps flush out toxins.

Kale. A member of the cabbage family, kale boasts a high content of vitamins A, C, and K, along with iron, essential fatty acids, calcium, magnesium, and potassium.

Mushrooms. Although a fungus rather than a vegetable, mushrooms have good amounts of niacin, folate, selenium, potassium, and phosphorus. It's better to eat mushrooms cooked rather than raw as they may contain high amounts of pesticides. Unless you are an expert, avoid picking mushrooms in the wild because some types can cause liver failure and death.

Peas. Although starchy, peas contain fiber and vitamins A, C, and K, in addition to folate, choline, calcium, iron, potassium, and selenium. In combination, these nutrients are thought to help reduce inflammation in liver cells.

Peppers. Incorporate all colors and varieties of fresh peppers into your meals. They contain essential fatty acids and vitamins A, C, and K, along with folate, calcium, magnesium, potassium, and phosphorus.

Spinach. This powerhouse leaf contains essential fatty acids and vitamins A, C, and K, as well as folate, calcium, magnesium, and manganese.

Sweet potato. A great alternative to the traditional white potato, the sweet potato offers many benefits, the most important of which is to provide fiber and reduce cell inflammation. Sweet potatoes also contain a large amounts of vitamin A in addition to vitamin C, folate, calcium, magnesium, and potassium.

Tomato. Versatile tomatoes contain large amounts of lycopene, omega-6 fatty acids, and vitamins A, C, and K, along with choline, potassium, and magnesium. Tomato consumption is especially beneficial for people with fatty liver disease and may also help reduce the risk of liver cancer.

Grains

An energy source, grains should be an important part of your diet every day. Remember, eat whole grains rather than refined grains like white rice, white bread, or regular pasta. Whole grains contain a lot of healthy fiber and proteins, as well as some vitamins and minerals. Don't restrict yourself to the common grains such as wheat, oats, corn, and rice. For added nutritional benefit and to spice up your diet, try the ancient whole grains that humans have been eating for thousands of years, including quinoa and farro.

Amaranth. The leafy part of amaranth is eaten as a vegetable, and the seeds are used as grain. Amaranth is gluten-free and the only grain with vitamin C. It is very high in protein and contains the important amino acid lysine. In addition, it contains iron, magnesium, phosphorus, and potassium. There is ongoing research on amaranth's potential to lower cholesterol.

Amaranth is very popular in South American countries and is sold, popped like corn, by street vendors. It is widely used in India, Nepal, and Peru as a breakfast dish. Try making it into a porridge, and top with fruit. Or add cooked amaranth to soups and salads.

How to cook it: Add 1 cup of amaranth to 3 cups of boiling water, cover and cook on medium-low for about 20 minutes, until the water is absorbed.

Barley. This versatile high-fiber, high-protein grain offers many health benefits—the major one being that it is heart healthy. In 2005, the Food and Drug Administration approved claims that barley can reduce the risk of coronary heart disease. The grain boasts high antioxidant levels and lots of vitamins and minerals. Choose hulled barley, a minimally processed form in which just the inedible hull is removed,

Most often used in soups, cooked barley can be substituted for rice and added to salads and other dishes.

How to cook it: 1 cup of hulled barley takes about 3 cups water or maybe more. Simmer for 45 minutes or so, check if it is soft, drain any excess water and let it sit for 10 minutes before eating or adding to recipes. Pearl barley takes 3 cups of water for 1 cup of grain and about 20 minutes to cook at a simmer.

Buckwheat. Despite its name, buckwheat isn't actually wheat but is related to rhubarb and sorrel. Buckwheat is gluten-free, has a high fiber content, and contains eight essential amino acids—and is particularly high in one of the amino acids, lysine. It is also rich in several B vitamins, phosphorus, magnesium, iron, zinc, copper, calcium, potassium, zinc, and manganese.

Buckwheat is the grain used in soba noodles, galettes (crepes), kasha, and buckwheat pancakes. The grain cooks quickly and can be used as breakfast porridge in place of oats or instead of rice in pilafs, casseroles, and soups.

How to cook it: Toast 1 cup of buckwheat groats in 1 tablespoon oil over medium heat, stirring frequently for about 3 to 5 minutes, add 2 cups of water, bring to a boil, then simmer for 10 to 12 minutes; once cooked the grains will still look moist.

Corn. Also referred to as maize in many countries, corn is believed to have been first cultivated by the Mayans and Olmecs, and then to have spread from Mexico throughout North America.

Pay close attention to the processing of the grain and the form in which you eat it. For example, avoid corn chips, buttered popcorn, and canned corn, and instead enjoy fresh corn on the cob, frozen corn (without cream or sauces), small corn tortillas, and polenta.

Farro. Farro has more fiber and protein than common wheat, and is particularly high in magnesium, zinc, and B vitamins. It's available in three types: farro piccolo (einkorn), farro medium (emmer), and farro grande (spelt). Don't confuse farro grande spelt with the actual grain spelt—they are completely different. You'll most likely find the emmer variety in the United States.

How to cook it: To prepare farro, soak the grain overnight. Then boil it as you would pasta for 10 to 15 minutes, and add it to soups for a grainy, nutty flavor with cinnamon undertones. You could even add it to salads for a pleasing texture and flavor.

Kamut. Kamut is high in protein (30% more than in wheat) and fatty acids, and contains minerals such as selenium (in considerably high amounts), zinc, magnesium, and manganese. It has a nutty flavor and is fairly chewy. Kamut is not gluten-free, so should be avoided by people with celiac disease; however, some people avoiding wheat products due to overprocessing of the grain, this may be a better alternative. In recent years, the grain has gained in popularity, and now it is added to soups and salads and used as a flour for baking.

How to cook it: Use 3 cups of water for 1 cup of grain; simmer for 60 minutes for a softer grain.

Millet. This gluten-free ancient grain from the Far East dates back nearly 10,000 years. India is the world's largest millet producer. In the United States millet is a major component of birdseed and is often wasted as a filler in bean bags. However, it has a mild sweet flavor, and its high fiber, antioxidant, and magnesium content offers many health benefits to humans.

How to cook it: Use 2 cups of water with 1 cup of grain and simmer for 20 minutes. Remove from heat and let stand for 10 minutes before serving.

Oats. Cultivated in Europe as long ago as 3,000 years, oats are popular in many countries because they lower bad (LDL) cholesterol and protect against heart disease. They also help stabilize blood sugar in type 2 diabetics.

Oatmeal is a traditional choice for breakfast in North America.

We recommend steel cut oats whenever possible. Even though it takes longer to cook, it has more benefits such as a higher fiber content and minerals content. Avoid heavily processed types forms of oats such as flavored oatmeal and baked goods that actually contain very little of the whole grain.

How to cook it: Use 3 cups of water to 1 cup of steel cut oats, bring water to boil, and stir in the oats. Reduce to low heat and simmer for 20 to 30 minutes, stirring occasionally. If the oats are still not tender and the water is all absorbed, add another ½ cup water and continue to cook for another 5 to 10 minutes. For extra protein, you can substitute milk for the water or use a combination of both.

ANCIENT GRAINS

Many of the grains discussed in this section have been cultivated for thousands of years. Quinoa was known as the "mother grain" to the Incas, and amaranth, barley, and teff have been around since the beginning of agriculture. Amaranth was a major food crop of the Aztecs (they called it *huauhtli*) and is believed to have been cultivated more than 8,000 years ago.

Barley dates back to the 14th century. Its prominence as a food in Europe during the Middle Ages was apparent when King Edward II of England standardized the inch as equal to "three grains of barley, dry and round, placed end to end lengthwise."

Also known as pharaoh grain, Kamut was discovered in ancient Egyptian tombs. When first introduced to the United States, in the early 1950s, it wasn't very marketable and ended up as cattle feed.

Another grain found in Egyptian tombs, farro has been a favorite of Italians for more than 2,000 years, It is believed to be the original ancestor of wheat.

Spelt is an ancient form of wheat originally grown in Iran around 6,000 years ago. It made its appearance in the United States about 100 years ago, when it was used as cattle feed.

Quinoa. Often dubbed a "super grain," quinoa is the only plant food that is a complete protein with all essential amino acids in a good balance. It has the highest level of potassium of all grains—important for controlling blood pressure. Quinoa also contains fiber and micronutrients such as manganese, iron, phosphorus, magnesium, zinc, and folate. Quinoa is very easy to cook; treat it just like rice. Prepare it as a pilaf, or as a main course with added vegetables. The white and red varieties of quinoa are readily available in stores. Black quinoa takes a little longer to cook than the white and red varieties. Caution: If you are taking certain diuretic medications, quinoa may not be a good choice. Ask your doctor about your potassium levels.

How to cook it: Use 2 cups of water for 1 cup of grain, boil, and then cook, covered, on medium-low for 15 minutes. Add ½ cup or so extra water for black quinoa.

Rice. This grain was first cultivated in Asia more than 4,000 years ago and is popular all over the world. It comes in many shapes and varieties, including brown rice, basmati rice, Thai jasmine rice, converted or parboiled rice, red rice, wild rice, and simple white rice, to name just a few.

Brown rice or basmati rice can be a healthy side dish. It is easy to cook and relatively inexpensive. Just pay attention to the portion size to avoid excess calories.

How to cook it: Add 2 cups of water to 1 cup of rice, bring to boil, and simmer for 10 to 15 minutes until all the water is absorbed; keep in mind that brown rice and wild rice may need more time, about 30 to 40 minutes. When in doubt, follow the package instructions.

Rye. Cultivated in Central and Eastern Europe since the Middle Ages, rye is commonly used as a bread grain in modern-day Europe. It has a high fiber content and lower gluten levels than wheat. Pumpernickel is a dark, dense bread made from rye. Pick up a loaf the next time you are in the bread aisle and try it in sandwiches or as morning toast.

Spelt. Nutritional benefits have spurred spelt's recent popularity. Although it contains gluten just as wheat does, it has more protein than wheat. It is a great source of calcium, magnesium, selenium, zinc, iron, and manganese, as well as vitamin E and niacin. Spelt flour can replace wheat flour in baking, and spelt pasta is readily available in stores.

How to cook it: Use 2 cups of water for 1 cup of grain, boil, and then cook, covered, on medium-low for 15 minutes.

Teff. This gluten-free grain has a high calcium content. It consists of 80% complex carbohydrate, which helps with blood glucose control in diabetics. You can cook the grain and sprinkle it over vegetables, or add it to soups and salads. In Ethiopia, teff is usually ground into a flour and made into injera, a flat spongy bread sold in health food stores.

How to cook it: For 1 cup of teff, you will need 3 cups of water. Bring it to boil, cover and cook on medium-low for 15 to 20 minutes. Stir. Remove from the heat and let it sit for 10 minutes before serving.

Wheat. This cereal grain originated in the Near East and now is grown worldwide. It is all around us in pasta, bread, breakfast cereals, pizza, baked goods, and many other foods.

Choosing to eat whole wheat products is the best way to include this grain in your diet. Processed and refined wheat has lost most of its nutrients.

LOAD UP ON HEALTHY CARBS

Here are some helpful tips on how to utilize healthier carbs in your diet.

Choose whole wheat pasta. It's a healthier choice than enriched pasta.

Opt for brown rice. It's much better for you than white rice.

Eat whole wheat breads. Choose whole wheat versions of sandwich bread, bagels, English muffins, and pita instead of white.

Try something new. Experiment with grains such as steel cut oats, quinoa, barley, and farro.

Think whole grain when baking. Substitute whole wheat or spelt flour for some of the all-purpose flour in a recipe.

Snack on fruits and veggies. Have one serving of a fruit or vegetable as your mid-morning snack, and another serving as your mid-afternoon snack. When you have a little more time, prepare ready-to-serve fruit and vegetable snacks and desserts. Prepare grab-and-go packages of fruit and vegetable snacks for work or school or to keep on hand at home.

Carry it with you. Some easy-to-pack fruits include apples, oranges, bananas, pears, berries in a container, plums, nectarines, and peaches.

Have some tasty fruit for dessert. Instead of eating cakes, pies, or cookies, grab a bowl of berries or sliced mango for dessert.

Processing gets rid of the most nutritious parts, the bran and the germ, which contain the most fiber and minerals.

Wheat berries. This is the whole wheat kernel (except for the hull), which contains good levels of fiber and iron. Cook in boiling water and eat as a cereal, or sprout the kernels and add them to salads. Wheat berries can also be ground into flour and used in baking.

How to cook it: 1 cup of wheat berries will need 3 to 4 cups of water. Bring to a boil and cook, covered, on medium-low for 30 minutes or so until soft.

Fat

Fat is the body's most effective way of storing excess energy. The liver is intensely involved in all aspects of fat metabolism, including breaking down the fat from food and then in distribution, absorption, and storage of fat.

It is important to choose healthy fat in the right amounts on a daily basis. Excessive fat intake leads to the storage of undesirable triglycerides, and a diet high in trans fat results in severe hepatic steatosis and steatohepatitis. In contrast, monounsaturated fat has been shown to benefit patients with non-alcoholic fatty liver disease by decreasing triglycerides. Studies have also indicated that inadequate intake of omega-3 and omega-6 fatty acids may promote steatosis and steatohepatitis, and supplementation with omega-3s has a positive effect on the liver.

If you wish to take fish oil as a supplement to add essential fatty acids—with the goal of improving heart health, boosting brain function, or relieving inflammatory pains—consult your doctor about the right dose. Avoid cod liver oil as its concentrated levels of vitamin A are harmful to the liver.

Oils

Oils such as olive, vegetable, canola, safflower, peanut, and rapeseed contain healthy fat, essential fatty acids (which are unlikely to deposit in the liver), vitamins E and K, and some potassium. Use oil instead of butter or margarine for cooking. You can also use oil in salad dressings and other sauces to add richness to dishes. A little bit contributes a lot of flavor. For people who need extra calories, oil is an easy way to add calories to their diets.

INCORPORATING HEALTHY FATS AND REDUCING OTHER FATS IN YOUR DIET

Cook with plant-based oils. Cook with olive, canola, or vegetable oil instead of butter or shortening.

Replace the butter in baking. Use olive oil or applesauce instead of butter when you bake.

Get an oil mister. It's a great way to cut down on the amount of oil you need for greasing or baking.

Look for less fat. Use low-fat or nonfat milk instead of whole milk. (Some liver patients may be advised to choose whole milk if they need the extra calories.)

Add nuts and seeds. Top salads, cereal, or vegetables with nuts such as walnuts, almonds, and pecans and seeds like sunflower, pumpkin, and sesame. In addition to health benefits, the nuts and seeds add crunch and flavor to your dishes.

Enjoy avocado. Add avocado slices to salads and sandwiches.

Choose oily fish. For a good dose of omega-3 fatty acids, put oily fish like salmon, herring, and sardines on your menu two or three times a week.

Make your own salad dressing. Instead of using store-bought dressings, make your own healthier dressing with olive oil, balsamic vinegar, and herbs.

Avocados

The avocado is a great source of healthy monounsaturated fat, which helps lower bad (LDL) cholesterol and improve heart health. It also contains a good dose of omega-3 fatty acids, great for vegetarians and for people who don't like to eat fish.

Nuts and Seeds

Not only are nuts and seeds a great source of protein, they also provide you with essential fatty acids. You can eat them as a snack or add them to salads and other dishes.

Foods and Nutrients That Claim to Heal the Liver

You may have heard or read claims that the following foods and nutrients help to heal or protect the liver. Read on to find out more about each substance and whether fact backs up claim.

Coffee

There is evidence that coffee is beneficial for the liver, possibly decreasing inflammation and scarring caused by chronic liver disease. Coffee consumption has been associated with reduced incidence of diabetes, cardiovascular disease, fat and scarring in the liver, liver cancer, and death from chronic liver disease. Remember, while coffee can help your liver, adding sugar to your coffee can hurt your liver. Coffee also has drawbacks: It can cause stomach upset, jitteriness, dependence, and withdrawal symptoms (such as headaches when you go longer between your cups of coffee) in some people. If you experience any of these side effects, you should cut down on or avoid coffee.

Milk Thistle and Schisandra

Extracts from these two plants are widely sold as "liver protective" supplements. While studies in animals and on liver cells in a laboratory have shown that milk thistle and schisandra can decrease damage to the liver from various toxic substances, studies in humans have not definitively shown a benefit. Milk thistle extract does not seem to be toxic to the liver. It may occasionally cause diarrhea and, rarely, nausea, upset stomach, or gas. Schisandra can cause heartburn, an upset stomach, and a rash, but has not been reported to cause liver toxicity. Avoid schisandra if you have a seizure disorder. As with all herbs and supplements, check with your doctor to make sure these extracts do not have the potential to interact with your other medications.

Wheat Germ

Wheat germ is rich in essential fatty acids, healthy fats, thiamin, niacin, folate, pantothenic acid, iron, magnesium, manganese, potassium, and selenium, which helps to reduce oxidative stress on the liver by aiding in antioxidant activity by protecting your body's cells from free radical damage.

Omega-3 Fatty Acids

Although some evidence suggests that omega-3 fatty acids reduce the amount of fat in the liver, no one yet knows the ideal dosage. Still, omega-3s are good for your health generally, so go ahead and eat foods rich in them: oily fish, chia seeds, flaxseeds, canola oil, walnuts, and eggs produced by hens fed greens.

Vitamin E

There is evidence that the antioxidant vitamin E may decrease fat and inflammation in some patients with non-alcoholic fatty liver disease. Talk to your doctor about whether taking a vitamin E supplement is right for you and about the risk of long-term, high-dose vitamin E supplementation.

Foods such as vegetable oil, poultry, eggs, whole-grain cereals, wheat germ, spinach, kale, broccoli, collard greens, nuts (especially almonds), and avocados contain vitamin E.

Adding Extra Calories to Your Diet

If you have decompensated cirrhosis, talk to your doctor and your dietitian about your caloric and protein needs. You may need extra calories (best in the form of extra fat calories) and protein to keep up. To help you add calories while staying healthy and not gaining undesirable weight or changing your lipid profile for the worse, here are some tips:

Use more olive oil. Drizzle it on vegetables, rice, and pasta.

Increase healthy fats. Use unsalted or freshly ground nut butters such as almond butter and peanut butter.

Choose milk instead of water. Make oatmeal and cocoa with milk rather than water.

Choose full-fat dairy products instead of low fat. You'll get the goodness of dairy with some extra calories.

Add full-fat ice cream or Greek yogurt to milk shakes. It will have the advantage of making the shake even thicker.

Add avocado slices to salads and sandwiches. Avocado contributes healthy fats and loads of vitamins and minerals.

Tips for Eating Healthy

Now that you know what foods to eat, the biggest challenge is sticking with your diet. Life can get hectic, so here is some advice to keep you on the path to good health.

Plan Ahead

When you're busy, it's easy to fall back into bad habits, like skipping meals, eating from the vending machine, and grabbing fast food or takeout on the go. Plan your meals for the whole week: breakfast, lunch, dinner, and snacks. See the worksheet on page 151. If Sunday is the day you have time to make meals with your family, then plan the meals, shop, and cook as a family. This is a great time to teach your family how to live healthy. Explore new foods and recipes with your family and friends. Form a cooking club. Prepare as many meals as possible at home from scratch.

Make some of the workweek's meals all at once, portion them out, and refrigerate or freeze them for quick healthy meals later in the week. To save time, make large portions of a single dish to have twice in one week, for lunch and dinner on different days.

Eat Healthy Snacks

In addition to preparing healthy, home-cooked meals, stock up on healthy snacks. Having well-timed healthy snacks between meals will prevent you from overeating, improve your energy level, and increase your metabolic rate (how efficiently your body burns calories).

Ideally, you want to have five or six small meals or snacks about 3 hours apart. It does not have to be an elaborate meal—it can be a yogurt, a handful of nuts, or a piece of fruit. When you go hours without eating, your body goes into starvation mode and decreases its metabolic rate to try to conserve energy.

If you plan to buy energy bars, do your homework by reading the nutrition facts panel and ingredients list before buying. Make sure that the energy comes from protein and complex carbohydrates (and not from sugar) with at least 4 grams of fiber per serving. Also be sure the bar is not high in sodium. On the ingredients list, look for wholesome ingredients such as nuts, seeds, dried fruit, and grains. If you see ingredient names that you do not recognize, skip to the next bar. Alternatively, you can make the trail mix recipe provided on page 112 and carry individual servings with you.

Keep a Food and Activity Diary

Now that you know what can be toxic to your liver and what is healthy for your liver, examine what you have been doing. Keep an accurate and detailed food and activity diary for a typical 2-week period in your life. Then go back and analyze your diary to see what is toxic to your liver and what is healthy for your liver. Highlight in one color the toxic items, and in another color the liver-healthy items. Keep the things highlighted in the color that indicates liver health, and change the things highlighted in the color that indicates liver toxicity. If there are areas you need to work on— such as drinking more water, increasing liver-healthy foods, or cutting out added sugar, sodium, saturated fat, alcohol, and other toxins—focus your energy in those areas. Changing your lifestyle is not easy, but making one change at a time makes it simpler and more manageable.

CHAPTER 6

PROMOTING LIVER HEALTH THROUGH EXERCISE

Our bodies were meant to keep moving. A lack of physical activity is one of the leading causes of preventable deaths in the world. It has been associated with increased risk of obesity, stroke, heart disease, type 2 diabetes, high cholesterol, high blood pressure, depression, certain types of cancer, arthritis, and falls.

How Exercise Promotes Health

You know you should be exercising. And it's really not that hard to work it into your daily routine. In fact, studies have shown that just 20 minutes a day of brisk walking reduces your risk of early death. The following are some of the ways that exercise can benefit your health.

Helps with weight loss and management. Exercise burns calories, which helps you lose weight and remain at a healthy weight. The more intensive and longer the exercise, the more calories you burn. Have you noticed that people who run marathons eat constantly yet are lean: It's because their running burns off an enormous number of calories. So treating yourself to a slice of birthday cake does not have to translate to weight gain. Go for a run and burn off the calories while exercising your heart, lungs, and muscles.

Prevents or improves high cholesterol, high blood pressure, and diabetes. If your doctor has expressed concern about your cholesterol, blood pressure, or blood sugar level, get moving! Regular exercise will improve those levels while lowering your risk of heart attack and stroke.

Decreases the risk of cancer. Exercise is associated with a lower risk of certain cancers such as breast and colon cancers. A study showed that the more active a woman is, the less chance she has of getting breast cancer. The same applies for colon cancer, for both men and women: Increasing physical activity can reduce colon cancer risk by up to 30% to 40%.

Decreases the risk of osteoporosis. Osteoporosis is bone loss that can put you at risk of fractures. Weight-bearing and resistance exercises help stave off osteoporosis. Weight-bearing exercises, in which your legs and feet bear the weight of your body, include walking, hiking, stair climbing, and dancing. Resistance exercises, in which you work against the weight of another object, include weightlifting and water aerobics.

Makes you think better! Exercise has been shown to help preserve brain mass and prevent cognitive decline as a person ages. It keeps your body and mind young.

Reduces the risk of falls in older adults. Exercise improves strength, endurance, and balance, all of which reduce your risk of falling as you age.

Improves mood. When you exercise, your body releases natural chemicals called endorphins, which bind to similar receptors in your body as morphine. They block pain receptors, decreasing pain and giving you a sense of euphoria, or a natural "high." That is why exercise has been shown to decrease depression, anxiety, and stress and to improve sleep. It also helps with chronic pain conditions such as fibromyalgia.

Increases energy. If you feel as if you are dragging all the time or can barely get through the day, that's the time to start an exercise program.

When you exercise, you are training your heart and lungs to work more efficiently, and you are strengthening your muscles. With regular exercise, you feel much more energetic. Just get started and keep at it. A few hours after exercising, you will fall asleep faster—and fall into a deeper sleep. So avoid exercising right before bedtime.

Improves sex life. Regular exercise is associated with less erectile dysfunction in men and enhanced arousal for women.

What Kind of Exercise and How Much

Now that you know why you should get moving, let's talk about how much and how often you should move.

Aim for at least 30 minutes a day. You can average it out over the week if you have to. If longer, less frequent sessions fit your schedule better, then go for it. Studies show that total amount, type, and intensity of exercise are key.

Intensity matters. Combine aerobic exercise and strength training. Aerobic exercise is exercise that requires your heart to pump oxygenated blood to your muscles, raising your heart and breathing rates to keep up the demand for oxygenated blood. Strength training is when you build muscle endurance and strength.

You should get at least 150 minutes per week of moderate-intensity aerobic activity or 75 minutes per week of vigorous-intensity aerobic activity. Moderate-intensity aerobic activity is an activity that raises your heart rate and causes you to break a sweat. It includes brisk walking, swimming, water aerobics, and doing household chores like pushing a lawn mower. Casually strolling in warm weather or riding a lawn mower does not count. Vigorous-intensity aerobic activity is an activity that raises your heart rate substantially, causes you to sweat, and makes you breathe hard and fast.

Examples are jogging or running, riding a bike fast or up hills, swimming laps, and playing basketball. If you are jogging at a pace where you can chat with your running buddy or on your phone, then the intensity is not vigorous. Push yourself to make your exercise count.

As you adapt to an active lifestyle, increase the amount of exercise you get. For even greater health, the Centers for Disease Control and Prevention recommend increasing the amount of aerobic activity a week to 300 minutes of moderate-intensity aerobic activity or 150 minutes of vigorous-intensity aerobic activity.

In addition to aerobic activity, get strength training—that's where you work all major groups of muscles, including legs, hips, back, abdomen, chest, shoulders, and arms—at least 2 days a week. Examples of strength training exercises are weightlifting, yoga, Pilates, heavy gardening, working with resistance bands, and push-ups or sit-ups (working against the weight of your body). To get the full benefit of the strength training, do repetitions of each activity. Usually, 8 to 12 repetitions of each activity count as 1 set. Do repeated sets of the activity until your muscles are too tired to do any more.

Exercise and Liver Health

Find something you enjoy doing. It doesn't matter whether it's running, bicycling, yoga, Zumba, dancing, soccer, or long walks with your dog. Just get moving!

Take advantage of every opportunity to be active. Park your car a little farther away from the store or your office, walk up a flight of stairs, or just take a deep breath a few times during the day. If you take public transportation, get on the bus or train one stop later or get off one stop earlier.

Set realistic goals. If you set an impossible goal, you won't follow through. Do something attainable. If you currently get no physical activity at all, don't aim to run a marathon in 3 months. You will set yourself up for failure. Start with a daily walk, and work your way up to 3 miles a day over the next couple months. Once you reach that goal, set your goal at speeding up the walk or jogging the 3 miles. Then increase the distance or speed.

Get a pedometer or activity tracker. Tracking your progress gives you something tangible on your journey to getting fit. Choose a model that is in your budget and feels comfortable. See the Physical Activity and Exercise Plan worksheet on page 155.

Motivate yourself with what is important to you. Chose a goal that's personal. Maybe you want to run a race with your teenage child or get off a medication, or perhaps you'd like to fit into your wedding dress or look your best for a school reunion. Post a reminder of that motivation where you will see it every morning.

Make a firm commitment. Designate a time for exercise, and add it to your calendar.

Make it social. Join a walking club, or make exercise a social event with friends. Get an exercise buddy and motivate each other. Set up regular exercise dates with your partner or other family members and get in some bonding time.

Try something new. Try a new type of activity to keep your regimen exciting. If you have never tried a dance class, sign up for one. If you have never tried swimming, take a class at your local gym. Trying something new will motivate you to stay physically active and not get bored.

Get a personal trainer. If financially feasible, work with a personal trainer for a few sessions and get some great ideas to target specific problem areas. Many gyms let you split the session with another person to cut the cost in half, and this way you will have a gym buddy for support and to keep you accountable.

Exercise at home. Depending on where you live, you might not be able to enjoy activities outdoors throughout the year. If that's the case, take advantage of exercise TV channels, borrow exercise DVDs from your local library, or use YouTube so that you can still exercise in your own home.

Please remember that if you have any existing injuries or are unable to participate in the types of activities described here, consult a physical therapist or exercise physiologist for an evaluation and safe prescription of exercises.

CHAPTER 7

JUMP OVER THOSE ROADBLOCKS

You now know how to eliminate toxins from your diet and your life, and how to incorporate liver-healthy foods. You have implemented changes to your lifestyle and set a new healthy routine: cooking and packing lunches and snacks, getting that run in four times a week, and making good lifestyle choices. You have more energy and feel great about being on the right path to a healthier liver and body.

To avoid being derailed, you need to be prepared for roadblocks that may come up. Certain situations can cause you to fall back into unhealthy habits such as skipping meals, overeating, making poor food choices, eating because of stress, not getting enough sleep, and not exercising. It's difficult to stay on top of things 24/7: cook your meals, go to work, exercise, get a good night's sleep, and spend time with family. Life gets in the way. Here are some common roadblocks you may face and how to get past them.

Busy Day

Thou shalt not skip meals! We have all been there: rushing to get the family ready and everyone out the door. Breakfast is the last thing on your list. Once you get to work, you start answering the 30 emails in your inbox. You work straight through lunch so you can make a deadline or get home on time. You don't have time to go to the cafeteria, but the vending

JUMP OVER THOSE ROADBLOCKS   89

machine is right outside your door. You figure that candy bar can see you through the afternoon until you get home for dinner.

Skipping meals causes your body to go into starvation mode. This leads to lower energy and a decreased metabolic rate as your body tries to conserve energy. You end up feeling more lethargic and less motivated or able to exercise. You are hungrier by the next meal, and that makes you overeat. So skipping meals makes you eat more in the end, burns off fewer calories, and slows you down. Ideally, you want to have five or six small meals (some of them snacks) a day. To get past this roadblock, here are some things you can do.

Plan ahead. Before your workweek, buy and pack a week's worth of breakfasts, lunches, and snacks. Lunch is easy. With every dinner you prepare, make a little extra and pack a few lunch-size portions in freezer-safe, microwaveable containers. Label the contents and date cooked. Stock your fridge and freezer with healthy homemade microwave meals. Grab one every morning on your way to work.

Make breakfast a simple and quick meal. Follow these tips for quick and easy breakfasts and snacks.

Breakfast

- Whole-grain toast or English muffin with natural nut butter
- Fruit smoothie with protein powder
- Scrambled egg, omelet, or hard-boiled egg (cooked the night before if you find yourself out of time in the mornings)
- Dry whole-grain cereal or low-sugar whole-grain cereal with unsalted nuts and dried fruit
- Hot cereal with fresh or dried fruit
- Snacks
- Glass of milk

- Veggies and dip (try cut-up peppers, cucumber, carrots, and broccoli with plain Greek yogurt)
- Fruit (easy-to-pack fruits such as bananas, pears, and apples)
- Yogurt with fruit such as berries, apples, and bananas
- Homemade trail mix (see recipe on page 112)

Traveling

A stressful business trip is coming up. Along with being thrown off your regular routine, you are stuck with a daunting drive or flight, hotel stay, business meals, and eating out. Here are some ways to bypass the roadblocks.

On the Road

Healthy eating options are harder to find on the road than at home. Unfortunately, it is impossible to drive an hour without finding a fast food restaurant with inviting signs and deals to lure you off the highway. The food at these restaurants tends to be high in sodium, sugar, and saturated fat. If you are hungry and have no other option, you might find yourself grabbing a bite. Healthy options are just as hard to come by at many airports.

Be prepared! Pack lots of tasty snacks ahead of time. Bring a cooler and fill it with healthy items like water or seltzer, hard-boiled eggs, sandwiches or wraps with whole-grain bread or pita bread, fresh or dried fruit, unsalted nuts, cut-up vegetables, and low-fat cheese.

- Your snack cooler will keep you full so that you can avoid unhealthy food on the go.
- If you forget to pack food or doing so isn't feasible, remember what you have learned about healthy food choices and portion sizes when you do stop for food. Many restaurants have nutritional information about menu items, so ask for it if you don't see it. If you choose a salad, ask for dressing on the side and only use a small amount.

Use a smartphone. There are smartphone apps to help you with food choices (see page 167 for a list). For example, many of the health and fitness apps such as MyFitnessPal and Fast Food Calorie Counter have menu items of restaurant chains in their databases.

The website HealthyDiningFinder.com lists healthy options from the menus of many restaurant chains. Its team of dietitians has analyzed the menu items of more than 400 restaurants and gives menu items designations such as "Healthy Dining" and "Sodium Savvy." Make sure to read their criteria for these designations.

If you are looking for snacks at rest stops, convenience stores, or the airport gift shop, some apps such as MyFitnessPal and Fooducate have a scan function. Simply scan the barcodes on packaged foods to find out the nutritional information. Fooducate will give you a nutrition grading as well. For example, nonfat plain yogurt or unsalted almonds get an A while chips range between C+ and D+.

Another helpful app called GateGuru tells you which restaurants are near your gate at the airport so you can evaluate your dining options.

Staying in a Hotel Room

If you are traveling for work, you will most likely be staying at a hotel. The same might be true when you travel for pleasure. There will likely be no kitchen in which to prepare food, and stocking up on a variety of healthy snacks will be hard. And you might be inclined to skip exercise. Here's how to keep yourself honest.

Take advantage of the mini fridge. If you can get a room with a mini fridge, then stock up on healthy snacks and breakfast items. Instead of grabbing a pastry, muffin, or donut on the go, you can have ready a healthy breakfast. Items to get for a quick healthy breakfast are milk, plain yogurt, fruit, washed and ready-to-eat vegetables (like peeled baby carrots), and low-sugar whole-grain cereal.

Stock up on healthy nonperishables. If you do not have a mini fridge in your hotel room, stock up on dried fruit, unsalted nuts, and fresh fruits that can be stored for a short time at room temperature (such as apples, bananas, and oranges). That way you won't go for hours without eating and arrive at a restaurant famished.

Make wise decisions at the breakfast buffet. If your hotel provides a breakfast buffet, make smart food choices. Avoid items loaded with sugar, sodium, and saturated fat. The typical buffet has some fresh fruit, hard-boiled eggs, nonfat milk, whole-grain cereal (without added sugar), and plain oatmeal. These are better choices then bacon, pastries, fried potatoes, and sugary cereal.

Pack your sneakers. Most hotels have a gym. Go on the treadmill for a jog. If there's no gym and you don't feel comfortable running outdoors in an unfamiliar place, do some simple exercises in your room. You'll find hotel room workout routines online.

Other Helpful Travel Tips

A vacation or pleasure trip can throw as many roadblocks your way as a business trip. Here are some tips on getting past those barriers.

Go for vacation rentals. We personally love staying at vacation rentals that come with a full kitchen. You can prepare meals and snacks at your home away from home. Even better, you eat when you are hungry and not whenever your schedule allows you to get to a restaurant. Apps like Locavore tell you which fruits and vegetables are at peak freshness where you are. Locavore also maps out the closest farmer's markets.

Do your own shopping when staying at a friend or relative's home. Ask permission to use some refrigerator space, and go food shopping at the local market. Your host will appreciate that you are trying not to impose, and you will win brownie points for offering to make a meal or two for your host.

Do some research. If you're traveling abroad, you might not be familiar with the local restaurants, cuisine, or local ingredients. Before you leave, research the restaurants and local markets so you can plan your meals.

Keep up with physical activity. Walk whenever you can. While sightseeing, this will allow you to take in more of the sights. If possible, take public transportation instead of renting a car. Plan some fun activities.

Eating Out

Eating out is associated with weight gain for many reasons. The average portion sizes in restaurants have doubled or tripled over the past 20 years. According to a 2012 survey, some 53% of us eat out at least once a week. We eat out because of time constraints or because it is enjoyable. You get to meet friends, catch up, and have food served to you without having to prepare it or clean up. So if you're going to eat out, do a little research beforehand. Look up the menu and nutritional information on the restaurant's website and on some of the apps and websites that track restaurant menus (page 165). Here's more advice on keeping control of your diet while dining out.

Avoid the bread basket. It's better to steer clear of an overflowing bread basket than to try and limit the amount of bread you eat.

Split a dish with one or two other people. Often, portion sizes are large enough that you won't feel deprived when sharing. You'll soon find that a smaller portion, if flavorful, is plenty satisfying.

Order an appetizer or a side dish instead of an entree. If you have no one to share a dish with, opt for one of these smaller dishes.

Take it to-go. Before you even dig into your meal, ask for a takeout container and pack away half or two thirds of it to take home. If you wait until the end, you are more likely to overeat. Order seltzer or mineral water with a slice of lemon. It's just as refreshing but much better for you than sugary beverages like soda, juice, or alcohol.

Clean up your salad. Tell your server to leave out croutons, olives, and processed meats from your salad. Also ask for olive oil and vinegar so you can dress the salad yourself.

Think grilled, steamed, or baked. If you don't see any of these options on the menu, choose a healthy protein like poultry or seafood, and request that the chef grill, steam, or bake it.

Hold the sauce. Look for options without sauces, which are usually loaded with sodium, or ask for the sauce on the side so you can use it sparingly.

Order an extra side of veggies. Choose an additional vegetable instead of a starchy or fried side dish.

Rethink dessert. Either skip dessert or choose fruit. If there is no fruit option and you still decide to have dessert, split a dish with other people—but avoid too much whipped cream, icing, toppings, and sauce. Alternatively, go for a latte made with nonfat milk.

Emotional Eating

You may have heard the term "emotional eating." Many of us have strong cravings for food when we are stressed, angry, afraid, anxious, bored, sad, or lonely. We turn to food for comfort, and that food is usually high in calories, sugar, and fat. Sometimes emotional eating can be impulsive or it can consist of bingeing, or eating a large amount of whatever food is around without even enjoying the taste. Often, an impulsive or binge eater feels guilty, which makes the person feel worse and more prone to repeated emotional eating. Here's how to get a handle on emotional eating.

Reflect and keep a diary. Think about your eating habits. Do you binge eat when you are feeling emotional? Keep a diary so that you can clearly make the connection between your emotional eating and its cause. If you find that stress triggers your eating, work on stress management with techniques such as breathing exercises, meditation, yoga, or tai chi. If anger is the trigger, work on managing your anger in healthier ways. If you are anxious, sad, or lonely, get support from friends, family, or a therapist. If boredom is the trigger, distract yourself by going for a walk, reading a book, or calling a friend.

Listen to your body. Before you reach for food in response to a craving, stop and listen to your body. Are you really hungry or is this emotional eating? If you are not feeling physical hunger, wait a little bit to let the craving pass.

Clear out. If you find yourself eating certain comfort foods during emotional eating binges at home, get rid of those foods.

Holiday Parties

We tend to eat more when we're with other people than when we eat alone. Often, we continue to eat even after we are full as we react to social cues. For example, even if you are full but you see friends at the dessert table telling you to try a piece of the amazing pie, you will indulge. The average American usually gains a couple pounds over the Thanksgiving and Christmas holidays. Most do not lose that weight gain, meaning that with each year the weight accumulates, leading to health problems. Here's how to avoid the hazards of holiday parties.

Have a healthy snack beforehand. Don't go to social functions hungry—that will only make you overeat.

Avoid sugary beverages and alcohol. If you are going to have a drink, limit it to one. Nurse it slowly. Drink lots of water and seltzer the rest of the time.

THE BUFFET

Say no to restaurant buffets! Avoid them. People tend to keep eating even though they are full because the food is right there in front of them. The food served is typically high in sodium, saturated fat, and simple sugars. And it's usually poor-quality food.

If you cannot avoid buffets because everyone in the group wants to go to one or it's the only option on a cruise or at a resort, here are some tips.

Use a smaller plate. People at buffets tend to fill their plates, so a smaller plate keeps you honest.

Check out all the dishes first. Before you put any food on your plate, see what's available and choose only the foods you really want.

Get one plate at a time. Finish one plate of food before you even think about eating any more.

Keep portion size in mind. Yes, you can eat all you want to at a buffet, but don't.

Drink lots of water. It will make you feel full so you don't eat as much.

Chew slowly. Make your plate of food last as long as possible.

Start with vegetables. The major portion of your meal should consist of healthy vegetables, so choose them first before filling the plate with other items.

Avoid foods you know are bad for you. That means skipping fried foods, casseroles, pasta dishes, and heavily sauced foods.

Choose steamed, grilled, or baked. Those are the healthiest options.

Minimize sauces, toppings, and marinades. If you decide to have any of these, take just a little bit.

Choose fresh fruit for dessert. Buffets often have fresh fruit right next to the decadent desserts. You know which one to choose.

Do not linger near the food table. You're more likely to keep eating when you are full simply because the food is right next to you.

Socialize. Talk and mingle between bites so that you are eating slowly and letting your body digest and feeling the fullness.

Use a small plate. Fill your small plate with vegetable dishes, lean protein, and whole grains.

Avoid fried foods and heavily sauced foods. If those are your only choices and you don't want to offend your host, take very small portions.

Stop and think. Before going back to refill your plate, stop and ask yourself if you are really still hungry.

Dessert? Yes, it's a special occasion. Of course, you are going to have dessert. But you're also going to run a few extra miles to work off the calories. Take a small portion if it's buffet-style or share a dessert if it is not.

PART 3

RECIPES FOR A HEALTHY LIVER

Now is the time to put into practice what you have learned about macronutrients and micronutrients, healthy portion sizes, foods for a healthy liver, reading food labels, and eliminating toxins from your diet. Make your meal plans using the worksheet on page 151 and the recipes in this book. These recipes use liver-healthy ingredients that provide you with fiber, complex carbohydrates, lean protein, vitamin- and mineral-rich fruits and vegetables, and healthy fat. They are heavy on flavor from herbs and spices, but low on sodium and sugar. Easy to follow, the recipes require a limited number of ingredients so they are not intimidating. Each recipe lists the total calories, protein, sodium, and saturated fat per serving. Keeping in mind that healthy eating does not have to be boring and bland, feel free to adjust the amount of spices to your taste.

If you don't already have them, consider purchasing a few basic items such as a blender (nothing fancy), pressure cooker, wok, saucepan, oil mister, roasting pan, and perhaps even a slow cooker. These few items will come in handy for many recipes and are well worth the investment. In the long run, you'll save money by eating in more often.

CHAPTER 8
BREAKFAST

As you have heard many times before, breakfast is the most important meal of the day, so try not to miss it! We have some simple, healthy ideas for you to make it easier to prepare the first meal of the day.

KAMUT PORRIDGE

SERVES 2

CALORIES: 435   **PROTEIN:** 16 g   **SODIUM:** 4 mg   **SATURATED FAT:** 2 g

1 cup Kamut

3 cups water (or a combination of water and milk for creamier consistency)

1 cup fresh or frozen berries

½ cup chopped walnuts

1 teaspoon ground flaxseeds

1 teaspoon chia seeds

1 teaspoon honey (optional)

1 Cook the Kamut and water in a covered pot over medium heat for 10 to 15 minutes. If using frozen berries, add them about halfway through; if using fresh berries, toss them in after the porridge is done. Add the walnuts, seeds, and honey at the end and stir into the porridge. Enjoy warm.

Variation
Substitute with 1 cup of chopped or sliced apples, pears, or pomegranate seeds for the berries.

TEFF "MEAL" WITH DRIED FRUIT

SERVES 2

CALORIES: 475 PROTEIN: 13 g SODIUM: 1 mg SATURATED FAT: 1 g

1 cup whole-grain teff

3 cups boiling water (or a
combination of milk and water
for a creamier consistency),
or more if needed

¾ cup chopped dates

½ teaspoon ground cinnamon

2 tablespoons honey

½ cup slivered or chopped almonds

1 Toast the teff grains in a saucepan over medium heat for about 3 to
5 minutes, stirring often to release a pleasing aroma. Add the boiling
water, and cook, covered, for approximately 10 minutes. Stir in the
dates, cinnamon, and honey. Cover and cook until the grains are
tender and have a porridge consistency. Add more water or hot milk
as needed.

2 Remove from the heat when completely cooked, add the almonds,
and enjoy.

RYE PORRIDGE

SERVES 2

CALORIES: 300 PROTEIN: 13 g SODIUM: 1 mg UNSATURATED FAT: 2 g

1 cup rye seeds

2 cups water

pinch of ground cloves

¼ cup chopped prunes

1 In a saucepan, bring the rye, water, and cloves to a boil. Turn the heat
to medium-low, and cook for 10 to 15 minutes until the water is
absorbed. Let the porridge sit for a few minutes. Top with chopped
prunes and serve.

Variation

Add ½ cup chopped apple and 1 tablespoon of raisins before or after the
porridge is cooked, depending on your preference.

BLUEBERRY OATMEAL

A high-fiber food rich in vitamins, minerals, and antioxidants, oatmeal is thought to lower cholesterol and high blood pressure, help with weight control, and reduce the risk of diabetes and heart disease. This blueberry oatmeal is a tastier and more colorful twist on traditional breakfast oatmeal.

SERVES 1

CALORIES: 350   PROTEIN: 16 g   SODIUM: 107 mg   SATURATED FAT: 1 g

¼ cup uncooked quick cook oatmeal or steel cut oats

1 cup nonfat milk (can be adjusted based on desired consistency)

½ cup fresh or frozen blueberries

1 tablespoon unsalted almond butter

1 teaspoon pasteurized honey

1 tablespoon ground flaxseeds

1 tablespoon chia seeds (optional)

1 In a small pot over medium-low heat, add all the ingredients expect the seeds. Let cook for 5 to 8 minutes, stirring occasionally. Remove from the heat, and stir in the flaxseeds and, if desired, chia seeds. Enjoy immediately.

2 As an alternative, cook the oatmeal along with the other ingredients (except the seeds) in the microwave for 2 to 3 minutes (or according to package directions). Remove the bowl from the microwave and stir in the seeds.

Variations

Use 1 tablespoon of unsalted peanut butter instead of almond butter

Choose ½ cup mixed berries, ½ an apple and cinnamon, or ½ a medium banana and 1 tablespoon of walnuts.

STEEL CUT OATS

Steel cut oats are a healthy alternative with more fiber, but they take longer to cook. Check the package for cooking times, but it usually takes about 20 minutes to cook steel cut oats on the stove, which produces a better consistency than cooking in the microwave.

OMELET WITH MUSHROOMS AND LEEKS

Kick-starting your morning with a healthy breakfast will fill you up and prevent you from overeating the rest of the day. This easy-to-make, high-protein dish is the perfect way to get your day going.

SERVES 1

CALORIES: 300   PROTEIN: 13 g   SODIUM: 108 mg   UNSATURATED FAT: 6 g

1 tablespoon olive oil	¼–½ cup chopped mushrooms
¼ cup chopped leeks	black pepper
1 clove garlic, crushed	1 ounce Swiss cheese, diced
2 free-range eggs	

1 In a pan over medium heat, heat the olive oil. Add the leeks and garlic, lower the heat to a simmer, and let cook for 3 to 5 minutes. Break the eggs in a bowl and whisk, working in the mushrooms and black pepper to taste.

2 When the leeks are slightly soft, add the beaten egg mixture and let cook until the eggs are cooked through, about 5 minutes. If you prefer a more thoroughly cooked egg, flip the omelet and brown on both sides. Sprinkle with the cheese and more black pepper if desired. Remove from heat and serve.

Variations
Substitute vegetables, herbs, and spices for a change of pace. Try:

Tomato and Basil: Sauté ½ cup of chopped tomatoes for just 10 seconds. Add ¼ cup of chopped basil and immediately pour in the egg mixture and follow the rest of the recipe above.

Peppers and Spices: Add ¼ cup of chopped bell pepper (red, yellow, or green), ¼ cup of chopped tomato, 1 tablespoon of fresh green chile, or fresh basil, chives, or cilantro.

For extra calories, use 2 tablespoons of olive oil.

SCRAMBLED EGGS WITH ASPARAGUS AND PEPPERS

Here is another easy way to cook eggs, and the best thing is that these eggs can be made ahead of time and reheated in the microwave or on the stovetop. You could also use this as filling for a small whole wheat wrap for lunch or on its own as a snack. Don't be afraid to cook asparagus—it's so tender and cooks fast when fresh. A combination of orange, red, and green bell peppers makes the dish so colorful that anyone will want to try it.

SERVES 1

CALORIES: 350   PROTEIN: 17 g   SODIUM: 177 mg   UNSATURATED FAT: 17 g

1 tablespoon olive oil

2 free-range eggs

½ cup chopped asparagus (about 4–5 spears), stalks removed

1 cup chopped bell peppers

2 tablespoons milk

1 tablespoon chopped fresh chives or 1 teaspoon dried chives

dash of paprika (optional)

a few shavings of Parmesan cheese

1 Heat the olive oil in a pan over medium heat. Break the eggs directly into the pan and scramble them. When they are semi-cooked, add the vegetables and milk. Cook for a couple of minutes, then add the chives and paprika. Before serving, add a shaving of Parmesan cheese for an extra kick.

CHAPTER 9
SHAKES & SMOOTHIES

Shakes and smoothies are easy to make, nutritious, and versatile. Have them for breakfast or as a tasty, satisfying low-calorie snack between meals to get plenty of fiber and protein. Smoothies don't always have to be made with fruit—you can use a delicious mix of vegetables to get your fill of fiber, vitamins, and minerals. For people with decompensated cirrhosis, struggling to meet their energy needs with solid food, smoothies are a great way to increase calories and protein by using whole milk and full-fat yogurt.

EXOTIC FRUIT SMOOTHIE

Taste tropical paradise in a glass! This delicious smoothie is packed with vitamins, fiber, and protein. Have it as a mid-afternoon treat or a healthy dessert. If fresh fruit isn't available, use frozen instead.

SERVES 1

CALORIES: 215   PROTEIN: 11 g   SODIUM: 152 mg   SATURATED FAT: 1 g

½ cup chopped pineapple

½ cup mango pieces

½ medium banana

½ cup low-fat plain Greek yogurt

3 tablespoons–½ cup milk (optional)

1 Blend all of the ingredients together in a blender. Add milk if you prefer a thinner consistency. You can add a few ice cubes if you like your smoothie cold.

Variation
Use coconut milk in place of cow's milk.

MIXED BERRY SMOOTHIE

Full of vitamin C, antioxidants, calcium, and protein, this nutritious smoothie is refreshing and super easy to make. It can be made year-round with frozen berries.

SERVES 1

CALORIES: 175   PROTEIN: 11 g   SODIUM: 130 mg   SATURATED FAT: 1 g

½ cup whole strawberries

½ blueberries

¼ cup blackberries

¾ cup low-fat plain Greek yogurt

3–4 ice cubes (omit if using frozen berries)

½ cup milk (optional)

1 Blend all of the ingredients together in a blender for a smooth consistency. You can add milk if you like a thinner consistency. Choose nonfat milk for fewer calories, or whole milk if you need extra calories.

FROZEN BANANA AND BERRY SMOOTHIE

The creaminess of the frozen banana makes this a perfect healthy summer treat that you can reach for instead of ice cream.

SERVES 1

CALORIES: 240   PROTEIN: 10 g   SODIUM: 120 mg   SATURATED FAT: 1 g

1 frozen banana (page 107)

1 cup mixed frozen berries

½ cup low-fat plain yogurt

¼ cup nonfat milk

1 Blend all of the ingredients together in a blender until smooth and enjoy.

Variation

Use whole milk for extra calories.

FROZEN BANANAS

If you have bananas that are overripe, don't toss them out—freeze them for later use in a delicious smoothie. Peel the bananas, slice into 1-inch pieces, and place on a plate or tray lined with parchment paper. Put the plate in the freezer for at least 1 hour, then transfer the pieces to freezer bags in single portion sizes (½ or 1 banana). Use a single portion in a smoothie.

CHOCOLATE ALMOND MOCHA SHAKE

What better way to start your morning than with this dairy-free shake packed with potassium and protein? The coffee (good for the liver) is a great pick-me-up, and the cocoa will satisfy your craving for chocolate.

SERVES 1

CALORIES: 165   PROTEIN: 4 g   SODIUM: 160 mg   SATURATED FAT: 1 g

1 cup unsweetened almond milk

1 frozen banana (see above)

1 tablespoon unsweetened cocoa powder

2 teaspoons instant coffee

1 Blend all of the ingredients together in a blender for a smooth refreshing cold treat.

Variation

For extra protein, add 1 tablespoon of almond butter.

COCO MANGO FRAPPÉ

Have this refreshing coconut water–based frappé filled with vitamins, potassium, and protein for breakfast, snack, or dessert. Also use it to replenish your electrolytes and cool you down after a tough workout.

SERVES 1

CALORIES: 360 **PROTEIN:** 16 g **SODIUM:** 400 mg **SATURATED FAT:** 3 g

1 cup coconut water (or more for a thinner consistency)

½ cup fresh or frozen chopped mango

1 medium banana (frozen for a colder treat)

¾ cup low-fat plain Greek yogurt

1 Blend all of the ingredients together in a blender and blend until smooth. If using fresh fruit instead of frozen, add a couple of ice cubes. If you prefer a thinner consistency, add as much as an extra cup of coconut water.

BLUEBERRY KALE ALMOND SMOOTHIE

This tasty powerhouse of a smoothie is high in vitamins, minerals, fiber, omega-3s, and antioxidants. Kale is low in calories and a good source of calcium and vitamins A, C, and K. The health benefits of flaxseeds have been recognized for thousands of years. In ancient Greece, the physician Hippocrates prescribed its use for intestinal ailments.

SERVES 1

CALORIES: 200 **PROTEIN:** 6 g **SODIUM:** 190 mg **FAT:** 4 g

1 cup tightly packed, freshly chopped kale, stalks removed

1 cup fresh or frozen blueberries

1 fresh or frozen medium banana

1 cup unsweetened almond milk

½ tablespoon ground flaxseeds

1 teaspoon pasteurized honey (optional)

1 Place all of the ingredients in a blender, and blend until smooth. If using all fresh fruit instead of frozen, add 3 or 4 ice cubes.

SPINACH SMOOTHIE WITH FRUIT

This flavorful combination of fruit and spinach contains protein, fiber, good fat, and loads of vitamins and minerals. It is naturally sweet, and the fruit disguises the mild spinach flavor. Always keep some grapes in your freezer—they come in handy for smoothies.

SERVES 1

CALORIES: 300   PROTEIN: 17 g   SODIUM: 223 mg   UNSATURATED FAT: 3 g

2 cups fresh baby spinach

½ cup frozen red grapes

½ cup fresh or frozen pineapple

1 tablespoon ground flaxseeds

½ cup low-fat plain Greek yogurt

1 Blend all of the ingredients together and enjoy.

CHAPTER 10
SNACKS & APPETIZERS

Here are some healthy alternatives to store-bought, pre-packaged snacks that are easy to make at home with healthy ingredients.

OATMEAL BALLS

Sweet, nutty, and filling, this snack is packed with fiber, protein, and omega-3s. It is the perfect substitute for a candy bar.

SERVES 7

CALORIES: 250 PROTEIN: 5 g SODIUM: 0 g UNSATURATED AT: 14 g

1 cup dry quick cook oatmeal

½ cup unsalted peanut butter or almond butter

⅓ cup pasteurized honey

1 cup unsweetened coconut flakes

½ cup ground flaxseeds

½ cup raisins

1 teaspoon vanilla extract

1 In a medium bowl, combine all of the ingredients. Cover and chill in the refrigerator for 30 minutes. Roll into 7 balls, and enjoy as a snack or dessert. They will keep fresh, in the refrigerator, for about a week.

MIXED BEAN SALAD WITH HOMEMADE WHOLE WHEAT PITA CHIPS

For parties, movie nights, or game days, reach for homemade bean salad and pita chips instead of high-fat, high-sodium store-bought chips and dip. Packed with protein, fiber, and flavor, this dish will satisfy your munchies.

SERVES 3

CALORIES: 170   PROTEIN: 10 g   SODIUM: 5 mg   FAT: 2 g

1 cup dried black beans, soaked in boiling water overnight*

1 cup dried chickpeas, soaked in boiling water overnight*

1 cup chopped red onions (about 1 medium or 2 small onions)

1 teaspoon freshly minced garlic

2 tablespoons chopped fresh parsley or cilantro

3 tablespoons fresh lemon juice

¼ cup chopped fresh tomatoes

2 (6-inch) whole wheat pita pockets

black pepper (optional)

1 If the beans are not soft by the morning, cook them over medium-high heat in a covered pot with fresh water until they are soft all the way through. Let cool. Mix the beans with all of the other ingredients (except for the pita bread) in a large bowl, and let sit for 30 minutes.

2 Cut the pita bread into small triangles with kitchen shears. Place on a baking tray, spray with olive oil, and sprinkle with black pepper if desired. Bake in the oven or toaster oven for 8 to 10 minutes at 325°F.

* Note that if the chickpeas or black beans are still hard in the morning, you can cook them in a pressure cooker with water for 5 to 8 minutes and they will be ready. If you don't have a pressure cooker, you can cook the soaked chickpeas or black beans, in a separate pot with plenty of water to cover them, over medium heat for about 15 minutes or so.

ROASTED ALMOND TRAIL MIX

This recipe is simple yet delicious. Roasting nuts at home is very easy, and making your own trail mix without the added salt and preservatives found in store-bought trail mixes is an added health benefit.

SERVES 6

CALORIES: 500   PROTEIN: 16 g   SODIUM: 5 mg   UNSATURATED FAT: 37 g

2 tablespoons canola oil

2 cups raw whole almonds

½ cup raw peanuts

½ cup raw whole cashews

¼ cup raw sunflower seeds

¼ cup raisins

2 tablespoons dark chocolate morsels (optional)

In a skillet, heat the oil over medium heat, and add the almonds, peanuts, and cashews. Cook until the color of the nuts change and you smell a nice aroma (about 3 to 4 minutes; keep stirring). Transfer the nuts to a bowl, and let cool completely. Add the sunflower seeds, raisins, and dark chocolate, if desired. Mix well and store in a glass container. This trail mix stays fresh for at least 2 weeks.

YOGURT DIP

A healthy twist on a traditional vegetable dip, this tasty version is loaded with protein, probiotics, and calcium, as well as other minerals. Dunk sliced peppers and chopped broccoli or cauliflower into the dip, or enjoy it on its own.

SERVES 2

CALORIES: 80   PROTEIN: 7 g   SODIUM: 100 mg   FAT: 0 g

1 cup non-fat plain Greek yogurt

½ seedless English cucumber

1 cup grated carrot

1 tablespoon chopped mint leaves

½ small chopped red onion (optional)

1 Place the yogurt in a small bowl. Wash, peel, and grate the cucumber using a cheese grater, then squeeze out the water and save it in a cup. Add the cucumber, carrot, mint leaves, and red onion, if desired, to the yogurt. Mix well. If the dip is too thick, add the reserved cucumber water to make it thinner.

2 Serve with whole wheat pita chips (see page 111) or raw veggies, as a side dish, or as a snack on its own.

Variation

Use full-fat yogurt if you need to increase calories.

CHAPTER 11

SANDWICHES, SOUPS, & SALADS

These are easy and nutritious recipes for lunch or dinner and are a much healthier, cost-efficient option for you than getting a store-made soup or sandwich.

ROAST TURKEY WRAP

Packed with lean protein and fiber, this delicious wrap will fill you up at work or home. Roast the turkey in advance on a weekend for an easy weekday wrap. This wrap is also a perfect way to use up leftover holiday turkey.

SERVES 1

CALORIES: 360   PROTEIN: 28 g   SODIUM: 328 mg   FAT: 18 g

1 tablespoon olive oil

4 ounces roast turkey, shredded (about 1 cup) (page 115)

1 small sprig of fresh rosemary or a pinch of dried rosemary

1 tablespoon dried cranberries

1 (6-inch) whole wheat tortilla or a larger one cut in half

1 cup baby spinach

black pepper or paprika

1 Heat the olive oil in a frying pan over medium heat. Add the turkey and the rosemary. When the turkey is slightly warm, turn off the heat and add the cranberries.

2 Place the spinach in the middle of the tortilla wrap. Top with the cooked turkey and cranberry mixture. Add black pepper or paprika to taste. Roll up the wrap and enjoy.

ROAST TURKEY

Roast a small turkey at home ahead of time. Slice or chop the meat, and save it in freezer bags for several meals (lasts up to 6 months in the freezer). This home-roasted turkey is much lower in sodium content than store-bought roast turkey. You can also roast a chicken using the same guidelines as below.

1 small turkey (about 6 pounds)

2–3 tablespoons of olive or canola oil

1 teaspoon of black pepper

slices of fresh lemon

chopped onion

cloves garlic

1 Preheat the oven to 350°F. Rub the turkey with black pepper and olive oil or canola oil. Leave it unstuffed to cook evenly, but add a few slices of fresh lemon, chopped onion, a few cloves of garlic in the cavity of the turkey for extra flavor.

2 Place the turkey on a rack in a roasting pan, and add 2 cups of water to the pan. Set the pan on the middle rack of the oven. Cook for about 12 to 13 minutes per pound.

Variations

Roast a chicken instead.

Toss all the ingredients (except the tortilla) with mixed greens.

EGG SALAD SANDWICH

Hold the mayo! This high-protein sandwich uses yogurt, which works just as well and provides calcium instead of fat. For a lower calorie and reduced-carbohydrate version, serve the egg salad on top of mixed greens. The egg salad will keep in the refrigerator for 3 to 4 days in an airtight container, so you can double the recipe and save half for lunch later in the week.

SERVES 1

CALORIES: 295   PROTEIN: 27 g   SODIUM: 340 mg   FAT: 11 g

3 hard-boiled eggs cut in small pieces (2 whole eggs and discard the third yolk)

½ cup nonfat plain Greek yogurt (or more for desired consistency)

¼ cup finely chopped celery

1 teaspoon Dijon mustard

2 slices low-sodium whole wheat bread or 1 (6-inch) whole wheat pita pocket

1 Mix the eggs with the Greek yogurt, celery, and mustard. Serve on bread or in a small pita pocket.

Variation
Serve on top of mixed greens instead of bread.

TUNA SALAD

Here is another variation on a classic sandwich filling: tuna salad without the mayo. This version is delicious, and you will love the texture and taste.

SERVES 4

CALORIES: 210   PROTEIN: 26 g   SODIUM: 68 mg   UNSATURATED FAT: 6 g

2 tablespoons olive oil

1 pound skinless skipjack tuna fillet (Bluefin or yellow are other varieties you could try)

1 cup finely chopped celery

¼ cup finely chopped red onion (about half a small onion)

2–3 tablespoons fresh lemon juice

½ cup sweet corn, fresh off the cob or thawed if frozen

¼ teaspoon black pepper

1 Heat the olive oil in a sauté pan over medium heat. Cook the tuna for 5 to 8 minutes on each side. Remove the tuna from the heat, and cut into small pieces. Pulse in the food processor, and set aside to cool.

2 Once the tuna is at room temperature, place in a large bowl and mix with the celery, red onion, lemon juice, sweet corn, and black pepper. Enjoy as a sandwich filling or on salad greens.

BABY SPINACH SALAD WITH VEGETABLES AND GRILLED CHICKEN

If you cook the chicken and chop the vegetables ahead of time, this complete meal takes less than 5 minutes to put together after work or a busy day of errands.

SERVES 1

CALORIES: 525   PROTEIN: 45 g   SODIUM: 250 mg   UNSATURATED FAT: 20 g

2 cups baby spinach

1 cup chopped red, yellow, and orange bell peppers

½ cup chopped broccoli

¼ cup thinly sliced white or brown mushrooms

¼ cup grated carrot

¼ cup chopped fresh cilantro

4 ounces (about 1 cup) grilled or baked chicken (page 132)

1 tablespoon raw or dry-roasted sunflower seeds (see below)

2 tablespoons Salad Dressing (recipe follows)

5 whole wheat pita chips, crumbled (page 111)

1 Mix together the spinach, peppers, broccoli, mushrooms, carrot, cilantro, chicken, and sunflower seeds. Toss with the dressing, and add the pita chips for crunch.

DRY-ROASTING NUTS OR SEEDS

Heat a skillet over medium heat and add your choice of raw nuts and seeds. Stir frequently for 5 to 8 minutes until you smell a nice aroma and they start to change color to golden brown.

Salad Dressing

This is a healthy and quick version of store-bought vinaigrette dressing. Stored in a glass container in the refrigerator, it will last for a few weeks.

SERVES 10 (ABOUT 2 TABLESPOONS PER SERVING)

CALORIES: 240   **PROTEIN:** 0 grams   **SODIUM:** 2 mg   **UNSATURATED FAT:** 20 grams

1¼ cups extra virgin olive oil
black pepper

¼ cup balsamic vinegar

1 Whisk the olive oil and vinegar together. Adjust the amount of balsamic vinegar as desired. Add black pepper to taste at the end and whisk again to make sure it's mixed in well with the oil and vinegar.

TOMATO SOUP WITH CHICKPEAS AND BLACK BEANS

This soup is filling because it's loaded with protein and fiber. You can double the recipe (minus the chickpeas and beans) and freeze the soup in small batches. Then add chickpeas and beans when you reheat a batch.

SERVES 2

CALORIES: 330   PROTEIN: 10 g   SODIUM: 84 mg   UNSATURATED FAT: 14 g

4 tablespoons olive oil

3 cloves freshly minced garlic

1 large onion, chopped

1 cup pureed carrots
(about 4–5 carrots)

4 pounds Roma or globe tomatoes, pulsed in the food processor

1 cup dried chickpeas, soaked overnight in boiling water*

1 cup dried black beans, soaked overnight in boiling water*

1 teaspoon fresh or dried thyme

½ teaspoon black pepper

4 slices avocado (about a quarter of 1 avocado)

5 whole wheat pita chips (page 111)

1 In a large saucepan, heat the olive oil over medium heat, add the garlic and onion, and cook for 3 to 5 minutes. Add the pureed carrots and tomatoes. You can add water for a thinner consistency if desired. When the mixture is heated through, after about 10 minutes, toss in the chickpeas and black beans. Cook until soft, stirring occasionally. You may need to add a little water to get the beans soft enough. When the beans are cooked through, add the thyme and black pepper.

2 Just before serving, add the avocado for a creamy texture and a dose of healthy fat. Crumble the pita chips over the top.

* Note that if the chickpeas or black beans are still hard in the morning, you can cook them in a pressure cooker with water for 5 to 8 minutes and they will be ready. If you don't have a pressure cooker, you can cook the soaked chickpeas or black beans, in a separate pot with plenty of water to cover them, over medium heat for about 15 minutes or so.

CLASSIC MUSHROOM BARLEY SOUP

SERVES 3

CALORIES: 130　PROTEIN: 2 g　SODIUM: 16 mg　SATURATED FAT: 1 g

2 tablespoons olive oil

1 cup chopped onion

1 teaspoon freshly minced garlic

1 cup diced carrots

½ cup chopped celery

2 cups sliced mushrooms

3 cups water

½ cup barley

black pepper (optional)

1 Heat the oil in a saucepan over medium heat. Add the onion, garlic, carrots, and celery. Cook until the onion is soft, about 4 to 5 minutes. Stir in the mushrooms, and cook for 3 to 4 minutes. Add the water and barley. Cover, bring to boil, and simmer until the barley is thoroughly cooked and tender, about 30 minutes. Before serving, season with black pepper if desired.

VEGETARIAN FARRO SOUP

SERVES 3

CALORIES: 400   PROTEIN: 27 g   SODIUM: 15 mg   SATURATED FAT: 1 g

2 tablespoons olive oil

1 medium onion, chopped

3 cloves garlic, chopped

1 cup dried chickpeas, soaked overnight in boiling water*

1 large carrot, chopped

1 large parsnip or turnip, chopped

½ cup dry farro, rinsed

2 cups water

2 cups chopped tomatoes

2 tablespoons chopped fresh basil or ¼ teaspoon dried basil

¼ teaspoon dried red pepper flakes (optional)

½ bunch kale, chopped, stems and ribs removed

¼ cup chopped fresh parsley

1 Heat the oil in a saucepan over medium heat. Add the onion and garlic, and cook until the onion is soft, about 4 to 5 minutes. In a separate pot over medium heat, add the drained chickpeas and enough fresh water to cover, and cook until soft, about 15 minutes. Add the carrot and parsnip or turnip to the onion mixture, and cover. When the vegetables are soft, about 5 to 8 minutes, add the farro, water, tomatoes, basil, and red pepper flakes, if using. Cook for about 15 minutes. Add the kale, which may need some extra water to help the leaves cook. Drain then add the softened chickpeas, cover, and cook for an extra 10 minutes. Serve garnished with chopped parsley.

*Note that if the chickpeas are still hard in the morning, you can cook them in the pressure cooker with water for 5 to 8 minutes and they will be ready. If you don't have a pressure cooker, you can cook the soaked chickpeas, in a separate pot with plenty of water to cover them, over medium heat for about 15 minutes or so.

CHAPTER 12
PASTA, RICE, & GRAINS

MASHED MILLET

You'll be pleasantly surprised by this spin on traditional mashed potatoes. Millet provides fiber and other essential nutrients such as phosphorus, manganese, and magnesium.

SERVES 4

CALORIES: 50   PROTEIN: 2 g   SODIUM: 0 mg   FAT: 0 g

1 cup millet

2 cups water

2 cloves fresh garlic, crushed

black pepper

1 In a covered pot over medium heat, cook the millet in 2 cups of water until the grain becomes thick and soft, about 30 minutes. Stir halfway through to make sure it's not sticking to the bottom of the pot. Once the grain is cooked, season with the crushed garlic and black pepper to taste.

Variations
Make this a breakfast dish by substituting 1 tablespoon of honey and any fruit for the garlic and black pepper.

WHOLE WHEAT SPAGHETTI WITH MIXED VEGETABLES AND CHICKPEAS

On a weeknight, you can get this nutritious, filling dinner on the table in less than 20 minutes. It gives you veggies, protein, and fiber all in one dish.

SERVES 2

CALORIES: 370 PROTEIN: 16 g SODIUM: 75 mg FAT: 2.7 g

4 ounces dry whole wheat spaghetti

2 tablespoons olive oil

2 tablespoons chopped or grated fresh ginger

3 cups chopped vegetables (fresh carrots, peppers, green peas, baby corn, and snow pea pods or standard frozen mixed vegetable medley)

1 cup dried chickpeas, soaked overnight in boiling water*

2 tablespoons fresh lemon juice

2 tablespoons chopped fresh cilantro

1 Cook the spaghetti in boiling water according to package directions (omit any addition of salt), and set aside. In a wok or saucepan, heat the olive oil over medium heat. Add the ginger, and sauté for 1 to 2 minutes. Add the fresh or frozen vegetables, and cook until soft, about 5 to 6 minutes. Toss in the chickpeas, and stir for a few minutes. Then add the cooked spaghetti, lemon juice, and chopped cilantro. After stirring for a couple of minutes, remove from the heat and serve.

*Note that if the chickpeas are still hard in the morning, you can cook them in the pressure cooker with water for 5 to 8 minutes and they will be ready. If you don't have a pressure cooker, you can cook the soaked chickpeas, in a separate pot with plenty of water to cover them, over medium heat for about 15 minutes or so.

BULGUR WITH MIXED BEANS AND VEGETABLES

A grain made from whole wheat, bulgur is high in fiber and rich in B vitamins, iron, phosphorus, and manganese. The combination of beans and bulgur provides the complete building blocks of protein your body needs. This is a perfect dish for vegetarians, but tasty enough to satisfy anyone.

SERVES 2

CALORIES: 330   PROTEIN: 13 g   SODIUM: 15 mg   FAT: 8 g

½ cup dry bulgur

1 tablespoon olive oil

½ cup chopped red onion

1 teaspoon grated or finely chopped fresh ginger

1 cup chopped tomatoes

½ small jalapeño, chopped (optional)

½ cup dried kidney beans, soaked overnight in boiling water*

½ cup dried black-eyed peas, soaked overnight in boiling water*

¼ cup chopped fresh cilantro

2 tablespoons fresh lemon juice

1 Cook the bulgur in boiling water according to package directions. In a saucepan, heat the olive oil over medium heat and add the red onion and ginger. Cook until the onion is soft, about 5 minutes. Add the chopped tomatoes (and jalapeño if desired), mix well, and cook for a couple more minutes. Add the kidney beans and black-eyed peas, and cook for another 10 minutes until the beans are semisoft. Serve over the cooked bulgur, add the lemon juice, and garnish with the cilantro.

*Note that if the beans or black-eyed peas are still hard in the morning, you can cook them in a separate pot with plenty of water to cover them, over medium heat for about 15 minutes or so.

PASTA WITH GREEN VEGETABLES

This is another way to look at pasta—as a vehicle for flavorful vegetables brimming with vitamins and minerals. A little pasta goes a long way in a dish like this.

SERVES 2

CALORIES: 500   PROTEIN: 20 g   SODIUM: 114 mg   UNSATURATED FAT: 15 g

1 cup dry whole wheat pasta such as penne or rotini

2 tablespoons olive oil or canola oil

½ cup chopped leeks

2 cloves garlic, finely chopped, or ½ teaspoon garlic powder

4 cups chopped spinach

1 cup chopped kale, stems and ribs removed

1 cup chopped broccoli florets

1 cup snow pea pods

pinch of oregano leaves

black pepper or crushed red pepper

1 Cook the pasta according to package directions (omit added salt), and set aside. In a saucepan, heat the oil over medium heat, and add the leeks and garlic. Once the leeks are soft, about 4 to 5 minutes, add the spinach and kale. Let cook for about 5 to 6 minutes, then add the broccoli florets. Add the snow pea pods at the very end, and remove the vegetables from the heat.

2 Serve the vegetable mixture over the pasta. Season with oregano and pepper to taste.

Variations

Complete the dish with baked chicken or cooked shrimp. For a vegetarian dish, add cubed extra-firm tofu.

MULTIGRAIN PILAF

SERVES 3

CALORIES: 300　PROTEIN: 8 g　SODIUM: 14 mg　SATURATED FAT: 1 g

1 cup millet, amaranth, or quinoa, or a combination of the three

2 cups water

¼ cup chopped green onion

¼ teaspoon ground cumin

½ cup chopped tomato

½ yellow squash, grated

½ cup finely chopped red bell pepper

black pepper

1 Toast the grain in a saucepan over low heat for 4 to 6 minutes, stirring occasionally and making sure not to let it burn. Let cool for a few minutes, add the water, and bring to a boil. Raise the heat to medium-low, and cook the grain until soft, about 10 to 15 minutes; refer to the grains section for individual grain cooking times.

2 In a small pan over low heat, combine the green onion, cumin, tomato, squash, and bell pepper. Once the vegetables are slightly soft, about 3 to 4 minutes, turn off the heat. Mix the vegetables with the grain, add black pepper to taste, and serve.

TOMATO AND BROCCOLI RICE

This recipe is a great way to incorporate several vegetables in one dish, and it's so flavorful that you won't miss adding salt. Serve this rice with chicken or fish.

SERVES 2

CALORIES: 250   PROTEIN: 5 g   SODIUM: 17 mg   UNSATURATED FAT: 7 g

1 cup dry brown rice or basmati rice

2 tablespoons olive oil

1 medium onion, chopped

2 cloves garlic or ½ teaspoon garlic powder

3–4 medium tomatoes, chopped

1 cup chopped fresh or frozen and thawed broccoli florets

pinch of paprika or black pepper (optional)

2 tablespoons chopped fresh cilantro

1 Cook the rice according to package directions (omit any addition of salt), and set aside. Heat the oil in a saucepan over medium heat, and add the onion and garlic. When the onion is soft, about 4 to 5 minutes, add the tomatoes and simmer until cooked, about 5 to 6 minutes. Add the chopped broccoli and paprika or black pepper if desired. When the broccoli is semisoft, after about 5 minutes (frozen broccoli may take slightly longer), remove from the heat. Add the cooked rice and the cilantro to the saucepan, and mix well.

Variations

Replace the broccoli and tomatoes with 1 cup of corn, pea pods, or finely chopped cauliflower.

For extra calories, top off with a dollop of full-fat yogurt.

WHEAT BERRY SALAD

SERVES 3

CALORIES: 290 **PROTEIN:** 23 g **SODIUM:** 83 mg **SATURATED FAT:** 1 g

½ cup wheat berries

2–3 cups water

¼ cup chopped green onion

½ stalk celery, chopped

8 ounces (about 2 cups) roughly chopped Roasted Chicken Breast (page 115)

2 tablespoons fresh lemon or lime juice

1 tablespoon olive oil

1 tablespoon honey

1 Soak the wheat berries in water for 3 to 4 hours, then drain. In a pot over medium heat, cook the wheat berries in 2 to 3 cups of fresh water until tender, about 30 minutes. Set aside and let cool completely.

2 Mix the green onion, celery, and roasted chicken with the cooked wheat berries. In a small bowl, whisk the lemon or lime juice, olive oil, and honey until smooth, and add to the wheat berry mixture. Toss to incorporate the sauce.

Variation

Try grilled shrimp or cubed extra-firm tofu instead of roasted chicken.

KAMUT SALAD

SERVES 2

CALORIES: 315   PROTEIN: 15 g   SODIUM: 51 mg   UNSATURATED FAT: 12 g

1 cup cracked Kamut

3 cups water

2 cups chopped spinach

2 tablespoons shredded
Swiss cheese

1 medium tomato, chopped

¼ cup chopped walnuts

1 In a covered saucepan over medium heat, cook the Kamut in the water for 15 minutes, then let cool to room temperature. Toss with the spinach, cheese, tomato, and walnuts. Serve at room temperature or cold.

CHAPTER 13

CHICKEN, BEEF, PORK, & FISH

As we discussed above, getting enough protein calories is vital to helping your liver heal and function properly. Here are some tasty ways to get lean protein into your diet.

GROUND BEEF WITH PEAS

SERVES 2

CALORIES: 600   PROTEIN: 39 g   SODIUM: 186 mg   SATURATED FAT: 11 g

¼ cup olive oil

2 medium onions, chopped

1 green chile, chopped

1 teaspoon chopped fresh ginger

2 teaspoons chopped garlic

8 ounces lean ground beef

pinch of turmeric

¼ teaspoon ground cumin

¼ teaspoon chili powder

1 cup fresh or frozen peas

1 cup chopped fresh cilantro

1 Heat the oil in a wok or sauté pan over medium heat. Add the onion, green chile, ginger, and garlic. Cover and cook until the onion is soft, about 4 to 5 minutes. Add the beef, turmeric, cumin, and chili powder. Cook on medium-low until the beef is well cooked, about 12 to 15 minutes, stirring frequently. Add the peas and cilantro, and cook for another 5 to 7 minutes until the peas have softened.

2 Serve with cooked brown rice or quinoa, or with baked sweet potato.

SHRIMP STIR-FRY WITH MIXED VEGETABLES

Shrimp is high in omega-3s and protein, and low in calories. It can also reduce the level of triglycerides (a type of fat in the blood that can make fatty liver disease worse). Use veggies such as carrots, green and red peppers, broccoli, baby corn, and snow peas, or try a frozen Asian mixed vegetable medley (without added sauce). Choose either brown rice or whole wheat spaghetti to complete the dish.

SERVES 1

CALORIES: 600   PROTEIN: 22 g   SODIUM: 540 mg   FAT: 27 g

½ cup uncooked dry brown rice or 2 ounces whole wheat spaghetti

2 tablespoons olive oil

1 teaspoon grated fresh ginger

2 teaspoons chopped garlic

4 ounces shrimp, deveined and tails removed

2 cups chopped vegetables of your choice

3 tablespoons lemon juice

chopped fresh cilantro (optional)

1 Cook the brown rice or whole wheat spaghetti according to package directions (omitting any added salt), and set aside.

2 In a wok or saucepan, heat the olive oil over medium heat. Add the ginger and garlic, and cook for 2 to 3 minutes. Add the shrimp, and cook for a few more minutes until the color is dark pink. Add the mixed vegetables and lemon juice, and cook for a few more minutes. Serve with the brown rice or whole wheat spaghetti. Garnish with cilantro if desired.

Variations

Substitute cubed cooked chicken breast for the shrimp. For vegetarians, opt for cubed extra-firm tofu.

QUINOA WITH GRILLED CHICKEN AND VEGETABLES

Quinoa is a grain that was important to ancient civilizations in the Andes. It is now considered a superfood because of its nutritional value. This superfood is cholesterol-free and an excellent source of complete protein, dietary fiber, manganese, potassium, phosphorus, magnesium, calcium, and iron. Because it is gluten-free, quinoa is a great staple for people with gluten allergies. We like the combination of chopped peppers and broccoli, grated carrot, and snow pea pods in this dish.

SERVES 1

CALORIES: 600   PROTEIN: 34 g   SODIUM: 55 mg   FAT: 35 g

½ cup dry red or white quinoa

1½ cups water

2 tablespoons olive oil or canola oil, divided

few sprigs of fresh rosemary or ½ teaspoon dried rosemary

4 ounces skinless boneless chicken breast

¼ cup chopped leeks or red onion

1 cup mixed vegetables of your choice

1 In a small pot, cook the quinoa and water over medium heat for 15 minutes, covered. Once all the water is absorbed, remove from heat and set aside.

2 Heat 1 tablespoon of the oil in a pan over medium heat. Add the rosemary and the chicken, and sauté until both sides are cooked through (about 4 to 5 minutes on each side, but depending on the thickness of the breast it may take longer). Set aside.

3 In a small saucepan, heat the remaining oil. Add the leeks or onion and mixed vegetables, and cook for 5 to 7 minutes, until semisoft. Add the vegetables and chicken to the quinoa, mix well, and serve.

Variation

For a vegetarian dish, substitute 4 ounces of extra-firm tofu cut into 1-inch cubes, or 1 cup of cooked kidney beans, for the chicken.

PORK CURRY

Garam masala is an Indian spice powder sold in ethnic and specialty stores, and sometimes in the ethnic or spice aisle of grocery stores.

SERVES 2

CALORIES: 600   PROTEIN: 36 g   SODIUM: 104 mg   SATURATED FAT: 11 g

¼ cup olive oil

1 cup chopped red onion

2 teaspoons grated fresh ginger

1 green chile, chopped

2 cups chopped tomatoes

8 ounces lean pork, cubed
(about 2 cups)

1 teaspoon garam masala

1 teaspoon ground cumin

½ teaspoon turmeric

½ teaspoon chili powder

½ cup chopped fresh cilantro

1 Heat the oil in a large pan over medium heat. Add the onion, ginger, and chile. Cook until the onion is soft, about 4 minutes. Add the tomatoes, and cook until soft, about 5 to 6 minutes. Add the pork, garam masala, cumin, turmeric, and chili powder. Cover and cook on medium-low or low until the pork is thoroughly cooked, about 20 to 25 minutes. Remove from the heat, and add the cilantro. Serve with brown rice or quinoa.

BAKED SALMON WITH INDIAN SPICES

Spice up your dinner with this dish. Serve the salmon—high in protein and omega-3s—with brown rice or quinoa and steamed broccoli or green beans for a complete, nutritious, and satisfying meal.

SERVES 2

CALORIES: 160   PROTEIN: 22 g   SODIUM: 400 mg   UNSATURATED FAT: 7 g

3 tablespoons freshly squeezed lemon juice (about 1–2 lemons)

1 teaspoon grated fresh ginger

3 cloves garlic, minced

1 teaspoon ground cumin

pinch ground turmeric

chili powder (optional)

2 (4-ounce) skinless salmon fillets

1 In a medium bowl, mix the lemon juice with the ginger, garlic, cumin, and turmeric and chili powder if desired. Add the salmon fillets, coating both sides with the marinade. Cover with plastic wrap, and leave in the refrigerator for 2 to 3 hours.

2 Preheat the oven to 400°F. Place the salmon fillets in a baking dish lined with foil, and cook for 15 to 20 minutes, flipping the salmon after 10 minutes.

Variation
Instead of salmon, you can use fillets of tilapia, scrod, or any other white fish. The cooking time will vary based on the thickness of the fillet. Check halfway through to avoid overcooked, dry fish.

TURKEY MEATBALLS

Try this great-tasting, fat-free alternative to your regular meatballs. These turkey meatballs are packed with flavor and protein. You can serve them on whole grain pasta, quinoa, or rice, or sliced in a sandwich with mixed greens.

SERVES 5

CALORIES: 113   PROTEIN: 23 g   SODIUM: 45 mg   SATURATED FAT: 0 g

1 pound lean ground turkey (look for 99% lean ground turkey)

1 cup finely chopped red onion (about 1 medium onion)

4 cloves garlic, freshly minced

1 teaspoon ground cumin

pinch of ground turmeric

¼ teaspoon chili powder or paprika (optional)

¼ cup chopped cilantro

1 Line a baking dish with foil, spray with olive oil, and set aside. Preheat the oven to 350°F.

2 In a medium bowl, mix the ground turkey with the rest of the ingredients until fully incorporated. Shape the meat into small balls, about 1 inch in diameter, and place in the baking dish. Bake for 25 to 30 minutes, turning the meatballs after about 15 minutes.

3 As an alternative, you can pan-fry the meatballs in a skillet for 10 to 12 minutes, turning them halfway.

TUNA CAKES

Tuna is high in omega-3s, vitamin B6, and folic acid, as well as being a guilt-free source of protein. Serve up these cakes with salad and quinoa for a beautiful complete meal.

SERVES 4

CALORIES: 160   PROTEIN: 6 g   SODIUM: 25 mg   FAT: 8 g

1 pound skinless skipjack tuna fillet

½ cup finely chopped green onion

3 tablespoons fresh lemon or lime juice

½ cup non-fat plain Greek yogurt

1 teaspoon freshly diced jalapeño (optional)

1½ teaspoons fresh thyme or 1 teaspoon dried thyme

1½ teaspoons fresh rosemary or 1 teaspoon dried rosemary

2 tablespoons olive oil or canola oil

1 Cut the tuna into small pieces and pulse in a food processor. In a large bowl, mix the onion, lemon or lime juice, yogurt, jalapeño if using, and the herbs. Add the tuna, and mix well to combine all the ingredients. Shape into eight 2- to 3-inch cakes about ½ inch thick.

2 Heat the oil in a skillet over medium heat, and sauté the cakes until lightly browned, about 3 minutes on each side.

Variation
Use salmon instead of tuna for an extra dose of omega-3s.

SPELT AND SPICY CHICKEN SALAD

SERVES 3

CALORIES: 375   PROTEIN: 40 g   SODIUM: 122 mg   SATURATED FAT: 2 g

1 cup spelt kernels

6 cups water

2 tablespoons olive oil

1 cup chopped onion

1 teaspoon grated ginger

2 teaspoons chopped garlic

8 ounces skinless boneless chicken breasts, chopped

1 teaspoon paprika or chili powder

¼ teaspoon ground cumin

1 cup thinly sliced red cabbage

1 cup grated carrots

¼ cup chopped fresh cilantro

1 In a saucepan over medium heat, toast the spelt kernels, stirring until browned. Rinse in cold water, and set aside. In a large pot, bring the 6 cups of water to a boil, and add the spelt kernels. Cover and cook on medium-low for 30 to 45 minutes until the spelt is soft.

2 Meanwhile, heat the oil in a saucepan over medium heat. Add the onion, ginger, and garlic, and cook until the onion is soft, about 5 minutes. Add the chicken, paprika or chili powder, and cumin. Cover and cook until the chicken is tender and cooked through, about 15 to 18 minutes. Place on a plate, and set aside to cool. In the same pan, heat the red cabbage and carrots for 3 to 4 minutes. Sprinkle on the cilantro, and toss the vegetables with the chicken and cooked spelt. Serve at room temperature.

CHAPTER 14
DESSERTS

BAKED PEACHES WITH DARK CHOCOLATE

Peaches were the favored fruit of kings and emperors in China thousands of years ago. On a special summer night, serve this beautiful dessert to company or have it on your own when you want to treat yourself like royalty.

SERVES 4

CALORIES: 140   PROTEIN: 2 g   SODIUM: 27 mg   FAT: 7 g

1 tablespoon brown sugar

¼ cup crushed almond biscotti

4 teaspoons olive oil

2 medium peaches

½ ounce shaved dark chocolate

1 Preheat the oven to 400°F. In a small bowl, combine the brown sugar, crushed biscotti, and olive oil, and set aside. Cut each peach in half, and remove the stone. Fill the hollow in each peach with the biscotti mixture. Place the peach halves on a baking sheet, hollow side up, and bake for 15 to 18 minutes until softened. (As an alternative, you can cook them in the microwave on high for 3 to 4 minutes.) Sprinkle with shaved dark chocolate. Let cool slightly so the peaches are warm before serving.

WHOLE-GRAIN ALMOND BARS

Almonds are rich in vitamin E, which has been shown to help people with non-alcoholic fatty liver disease. The nuts are also a great source of protein, fiber, B vitamins, essential minerals, and good fat that can lower bad (LDL) cholesterol. This sweet, healthy dessert combining almonds as well as almond butter with high-fiber, whole-grain Weetabix will make you wonder why you ever settled for Rice Krispie treats.

SERVES 24

CALORIES: 80   PROTEIN: 2 g   SODIUM: 35 mg   FAT: 4 g

3 tablespoons almond butter

1½ cups brown rice syrup

12 Weetabix whole-grain cereal biscuits, crumbled

1 cup chopped unsalted roasted almonds

1 In a large microwave-safe bowl, heat the almond butter and brown rice syrup in the microwave on high for 3 minutes, stirring after 2 minutes. After the full 3 minutes, stir again until smooth. If using the stovetop instead, heat the brown rice syrup in a pot over low heat, stirring until the syrup is a liquid. Add the almond butter, and continue to stir until smooth. Remove from the heat.

2 Add the Weetabix cereal biscuits and chopped almonds to the almond butter and brown rice syrup mixture, and stir well. Coat a 13 x 9 x 2-inch pan with cooking spray. Using wax paper, evenly press the Weetabix mixture into the pan. Allow to cool, about 20 minutes. Cut into 2-inch squares.

FROZEN CHOCOLATE-COVERED BANANAS

These frozen chocolate banana ice pops are packed with antioxidants, potassium, vitamin B6, and manganese. They taste like decadent summer treats but are guilt-free.

SERVES 4

CALORIES: 240 PROTEIN: 5 g SODIUM: 10 mg FAT: 13 g

2 medium ripe but firm bananas

4 ounces chopped dark chocolate

½ cup chopped unsalted roasted almonds (optional)

1 Line a baking sheet with nonstick foil or parchment paper. Cut the bananas in half horizontally, and insert a stick into each half to make four ice pops. Place them on the baking sheet and freeze for 15 minutes.

2 Melt the chocolate in a double boiler, or in a glass or metal bowl secured over a saucepan of water, making sure that the bottom of the bowl does not touch the water. Once the chocolate begins to melt, stir it gently with a plastic or silicone spatula. When almost all of the chocolate is melted, set the bowl or top of the double boiler aside. Keep stirring until the chocolate is smooth and completely melted. As an alternative to melting the chocolate on the stovetop, you can melt it in a microwave-safe dish in the microwave, checking and stirring every 30 seconds, until smooth.

3 Drizzle each banana ice pop with the melted chocolate, then quickly sprinkle with chopped almonds if using. Place the ice pops back in the freezer, and freeze until the chocolate sets, about 30 minutes. The pops will keep in an airtight container in the freezer for up to a week.

RICE PUDDING

SERVES 2

CALORIES: 400   PROTEIN: 23 g   SODIUM: 174 mg   UNSATURATED FAT: 9 g

2 cups low-fat milk

1 cup dry white rice

1 beaten egg

1 teaspoon vanilla extract

dash of ground nutmeg

¼ cup shelled pistachios
or slivered almonds

few strands of saffron (optional)

1 In a saucepan, bring the milk to a boil, and then lower the heat to
medium. Add the rice, and cook until soft, about 10 to 12 minutes.
Stir in the beaten egg, and cook over low heat until the consistency is
creamy, about 3 to 5 minutes. Remove from the heat, and stir in the
vanilla, nutmeg, nuts, and saffron if using. Serve warm or chilled.

Variation

Use whole milk if you need the extra calories.

For a different flavor, add dried fruit such as raisins or cherries, or both.

BUCKWHEAT PORRIDGE

SERVES 2

CALORIES: 500   PROTEIN: 19 g   SODIUM: 109 mg   SATURATED FAT: 3 g

1 cup buckwheat groats

2 tablespoons raisins

1½ cups low-fat milk (or more for a smoother consistency)

2 medium bananas

2 tablespoons raw cocoa powder

1 tablespoon honey (optional)

1 Soak the buckwheat and raisins in the milk in the refrigerator for a couple of hours. In a food processor, blend the buckwheat mixture with the bananas and cocoa. You can add more milk if prefer a smoother consistency. Add honey if desired, and blend for another few seconds to mix well.

APPENDIX

Use these worksheets to help you stay organized.

Grocery Lists

Pantry Essentials

❑ Garlic

❑ Onions

Grains

❑ Amaranth

❑ Barley (preferably hulled)

❑ Brown rice

❑ Buckwheat

❑ Farro

❑ Kamut

❑ Millet

❑ Oats, steel cut or rolled

❑ Quinoa

❑ Rye bread

❑ Spelt

❑ Teff

❑ Wheatberries

❑ Whole wheat bread

❑ Whole wheat pasta

❑ Whole wheat pita bread

Legumes, dried

❑ Black beans

❑ Chickpeas

❑ Kidney beans

❑ Lentils (all colors)

❑ Pinto beans

Herbs, dried

❑ Basil

❑ Cilantro

❑ Oregano

❑ Parsley

Spices, dried

❑ Cinnamon

❑ Cumin

❑ Ginger

❑ Nutmeg

❑ Paprika

Pureed vegetables

❑ Butternut squash (comes in Tetra Paks, or cardboard containers)

❑ Pumpkin (usually comes in a box) without added sodium (check the ingredients on the label)

Fruit, dried

❑ Apricots

❑ Mangos

❑ Prunes

❑ Raisins

Nuts

❑ Dry-roasted, unsalted

❑ Raw, unsalted

Freezer Staples

❑ Bread: whole-grain breads such as sliced sandwich bread, bagels, and pita

❑ Chicken breasts

❑ Fish fillets: such as salmon, haddock, and tuna

❑ Fruit, frozen: Mixed berries, pineapple, mangoes, grapes, and bananas

❑ Ground turkey

❑ Herbs, frozen: such as cilantro, basil, garlic, and mint

❑ Vegetables, frozen: any variety without added sauces

Refrigerator Staples

❏ Eggs: free-range

Dairy Products (choose the percentage of fat right for your health)

❏ Cottage cheese

❏ Greek yogurt

❏ Milk

Vegetables (cut ahead of time and stored in airtight containers if desired)

❏ Broccoli

❏ Carrots

❏ Cauliflower

❏ Celery

❏ Cucumbers

❏ Green beans

❏ Spicy green chiles such as seranos, jalapeños, and Thai

❏ Peppers

Dark leafy greens

❏ Bok choi

❏ Chard

❏ Kale

❏ Mustard greens

❏ Spinach

Salad mix (washed and dried with paper towels, and stored in airtight containers)

❏ Butter lettuce

❏ Leeks

❏ Radicchio

❏ Red leaf lettuce

❏ Romaine lettuce

Herbs, fresh

❏ Cilantro

❏ Mint

❏ Parsley

❏ Thyme

Fruits, fresh (washed, chopped, and packaged in individual portions for convenience)

❏ Apples

❏ Bananas

❏ Berries

❏ Lemons

❏ Limes

❏ Oranges

Sample Meal Plan

Here is a sample 2-week meal plan including breakfast, lunch, dinner, and snacks. This plan includes many recipes from the book. We added more time-consuming recipes on the weekends when most people have time to prepare meals. We recommend doubling or tripling a recipe and freezing individual portions for lunch and dinner later in the week. Adapt the plan to your schedule. If you have more time on other days to prepare meals, do it then.

Sample Meal Plan: Week 1

	MEAL	MENU
SATURDAY	BREAKFAST	Scrambled Eggs with Asparagus and Peppers (page 104) Nonfat plain yogurt with bananas
	LUNCH	Roast Turkey Wrap (page 114) Apple Nonfat milk
	DINNER	Quinoa with Grilled Chicken and Vegetables (page 132)
	SNACK	Whole Wheat Pita Chips (page 111) Yogurt Dip (page 113) Chocolate Almond Mocha Shake (page 107)
SUNDAY	BREAKFAST	Omelet with Mushrooms and Leeks (page 103) Nonfat plain yogurt with fresh mixed berries
	LUNCH	Baby Spinach Salad with Vegetables and Grilled Chicken (page 117) Nonfat milk
	DINNER	Shrimp Stir-Fry with Mixed Vegetables (page 131) over brown rice
	SNACK	Oatmeal Ball (page 110) Coco Mango Frappé (page 108)

Sample Meal Plan: Week 1

	MEAL	MENU
MONDAY	BREAKFAST	Blueberry Oatmeal (page 102)
	LUNCH	Egg Salad Sandwich (page 116) Orange Nonfat milk
	DINNER	Baked Salmon with Indian Spices (page 134) Brown rice served with a side of stir-fried vegetables; cook using the recipe for Shrimp Stir-Fry with Mixed Vegetables but leave out the shrimp to make this a side dish (page 131)
	SNACK	Apple Whole Wheat Pita Chips (page 111) Leftover Yogurt Dip (page 113) from Saturday
TUESDAY	BREAKFAST	Mixed Berry Smoothie (page 106)
	LUNCH	Leftover Quinoa with Grilled Chicken and Vegetables (page 132) from Saturday Nonfat milk
	DINNER	Whole Wheat Spaghetti with Mixed Vegetables and Chickpeas (page 123) Turkey Meatballs (page 135)
	SNACK	Oatmeal Ball (page 110) Nonfat plain yogurt with banana
WEDNESDAY	BREAKFAST	Oatmeal with apples and cinnamon (page 102)
	LUNCH	Leftover Shrimp Stir-Fry with Mixed Vegetables (page 131) from Sunday over brown rice Nonfat milk
	DINNER	Tomato and Broccoli Rice (page 127) Grilled chicken breast; make the chicken breast according to the recipe in Quinoa with Grilled Chicken and Vegetables (page 132)
	SNACK	Almonds Orange

Sample Meal Plan: Week 1

	MEAL	MENU
THURSDAY	BREAKFAST	Frozen Banana and Berry Smoothie (page 106)
	LUNCH	Baked Salmon with Indian Spices (page 134) Brown rice Leftover stir-fried vegetables from Monday Nonfat milk
	DINNER	Pasta with Green Vegetables (page 125) Turkey Meatballs (page 135)
	SNACK	Nonfat plain yogurt with dried fruit Apple
FRIDAY	BREAKFAST	Oatmeal with Bananas and Walnuts (page 102)
	LUNCH	Leftover Whole Wheat Spaghetti with Mixed Vegetables and Chickpeas (page 123) from Tuesday Leftover Turkey Meatballs (page 135) from Tuesday Nonfat milk
	DINNER	Bulgur with Mixed Beans and Vegetables (page 124) Tuna Cake (page 136)
	SNACK	Orange Whole Wheat Pita Chips (page 111) Yogurt Dip (page 113)

Sample Meal Plan: Week 2

	MEAL	MENU
SATURDAY	BREAKFAST	Omelet with Tomato and Basil (page 103) Whole wheat toast Fresh fruit
	LUNCH	Tomato Soup with Chickpeas and Black Beans (page 119) Whole wheat pita bread Nonfat milk
	DINNER	Pasta with Green Vegetables and Cooked Shrimp (page 125)
	SNACK	Whole-Grain Almond Bar (page 139) Nonfat plain yogurt with fresh berries

Sample Meal Plan: Week 2

	MEAL	MENU
SUNDAY	BREAKFAST	Kamut Porridge (page 100) Fresh fruit
	LUNCH	Tuna Salad sandwich (page 116) Nonfat milk
	DINNER	Tomato and Broccoli Rice (page 127) Baked Tilapia with Indian Spices (page 134)
	SNACK	Roasted Almond Trail Mix (page 112) Nonfat plain yogurt with banana
MONDAY	BREAKFAST	Blueberry Kale Almond Smoothie (page 108)
	LUNCH	Roast Turkey Wrap (page 114) Apple Nonfat milk
	DINNER	Leftover Tomato and Broccoli Rice (page 127) from Wednesday Leftover grilled chicken breast from Wednesday
	SNACK	Apple Nonfat plain yogurt with banana
TUESDAY	BREAKFAST	Oatmeal with Strawberries (page 102)
	LUNCH	Leftover Pasta with Green Vegetables (page 125) from Thursday Leftover Turkey Meatballs (page 135) from Thursday Nonfat milk
	DINNER	Ground Beef with Peas served with cooked brown rice (page 130) Nonfat milk
	SNACK	Whole Grain Almond Bar (page 139) Orange
WEDNESDAY	BREAKFAST	Frozen Banana and Berry Smoothie (page 106)
	LUNCH	Egg Salad Sandwich (page 116) Fruit salad Nonfat milk
	DINNER	Stir-Fry with Mixed Vegetables (page 131) over brown rice
	SNACK	Apple Nonfat plain yogurt with dried fruit

Sample Meal Plan: Week 2

	MEAL	MENU
THURSDAY	BREAKFAST	Oatmeal with Mixed Berries (page 102)
	LUNCH	Leftover Tomato and Broccoli Rice (page 127) from Sunday
		Leftover Baked Tilapia with Indian Spices (page 134) from Sunday
		Nonfat milk
	DINNER	Pasta with Green Vegetables and Tofu (page 125)
	SNACK	Roasted Almond Trail Mix (page 112)
		Banana
FRIDAY	BREAKFAST	Exotic Fruit Smoothie (page 105)
	LUNCH	Leftover Bulgur with Mixed Beans and Vegetables (page 124) from last Friday
		Leftover Tuna Cake (page 136) from last Friday
		Nonfat milk
	DINNER	Baby Spinach Salad with Vegetables and Grilled Chicken (page 117)
		Leftover Tomato and Broccoli Rice (page 127) from Sunday
	SNACK	Whole Wheat Pita Chips (page 111)
		Yogurt Dip (page 113)
		Almonds

Meal Planning Worksheet

Put to work what you have learned and make your meal plan. Remember to avoid added sugar, sodium, and unhealthy fat. Create meals that, each day, include at least 6 to 7 servings of fruits and vegetables, 5 servings of complex carbohydrates, 3 servings of protein, and 3 servings of dairy products. Make extra portions and freeze them for days you know you will be too busy to cook.

	MEAL	MENU
SATURDAY	BREAKFAST	
	LUNCH	
	DINNER	
	SNACK	
SUNDAY	BREAKFAST	
	LUNCH	
	DINNER	
	SNACK	

	MEAL	MENU
MONDAY	BREAKFAST	
	LUNCH	
	DINNER	
	SNACK	
TUESDAY	BREAKFAST	
	LUNCH	
	DINNER	
	SNACK	
WEDNESDAY	BREAKFAST	
	LUNCH	
	DINNER	
	SNACK	

	MEAL	MENU
THURSDAY	BREAKFAST	
	LUNCH	
	DINNER	
	SNACK	
FRIDAY	BREAKFAST	
	LUNCH	
	DINNER	
	SNACK	

Water Intake Log

Mark each circle for every 8 ounces of water you drink.

DATE	WATER INTAKE (8 OUNCES EACH)
	①②③④⑤⑥⑦⑧ Yay! ⑨⑩⑪⑫
	①②③④⑤⑥⑦⑧ Yay! ⑨⑩⑪⑫
	①②③④⑤⑥⑦⑧ Yay! ⑨⑩⑪⑫
	①②③④⑤⑥⑦⑧ Yay! ⑨⑩⑪⑫
	①②③④⑤⑥⑦⑧ Yay! ⑨⑩⑪⑫
	①②③④⑤⑥⑦⑧ Yay! ⑨⑩⑪⑫
	①②③④⑤⑥⑦⑧ Yay! ⑨⑩⑪⑫
	①②③④⑤⑥⑦⑧ Yay! ⑨⑩⑪⑫
	①②③④⑤⑥⑦⑧ Yay! ⑨⑩⑪⑫
	①②③④⑤⑥⑦⑧ Yay! ⑨⑩⑪⑫
	①②③④⑤⑥⑦⑧ Yay! ⑨⑩⑪⑫
	①②③④⑤⑥⑦⑧ Yay! ⑨⑩⑪⑫
	①②③④⑤⑥⑦⑧ Yay! ⑨⑩⑪⑫
	①②③④⑤⑥⑦⑧ Yay! ⑨⑩⑪⑫
	①②③④⑤⑥⑦⑧ Yay! ⑨⑩⑪⑫
	①②③④⑤⑥⑦⑧ Yay! ⑨⑩⑪⑫
	①②③④⑤⑥⑦⑧ Yay! ⑨⑩⑪⑫
	①②③④⑤⑥⑦⑧ Yay! ⑨⑩⑪⑫
	①②③④⑤⑥⑦⑧ Yay! ⑨⑩⑪⑫

Physical Activity and Exercise Plan

Make a physical activity and exercise plan. Incorporate at least 2 days of strength training and at least 150 minutes of moderate-intensity aerobic exercise per week (or 75 minutes of vigorous-intensity aerobic exercise per week). Remember, moderate-intensity aerobic activities raise your heart rate and make you sweat. Vigorous-intensity aerobic activities raise your heart rate and make you breathe hard and fast.

Sample Exercise Plan

	DATE	ACTIVITY	DURATION (MINUTES)	AEROBIC OR STRENGTH?	INTENSITY
MON		3-mile run at 6 miles/hour	30 minutes	aerobic	vigorous
TUES		Rest			
WED		Lifting weights	60 minutes	strength	
THU		Rest			
FRI		3-mile run at 6 miles/hour	30 minutes	aerobic	vigorous
SAT		Yoga	75 minutes	strength	
SUN		2-mile run at 6 miles/hour	20 minutes	aerobic	vigorous
TOTAL	Strength: number of days **2**		Aerobic: number of minutes **80 min**		

Physical Exercise/Activity Log

	DATE	ACTIVITY	DURATION (MINUTES)	AEROBIC OR STRENGTH?	INTENSITY
MONDAY					
TUESDAY					
WEDNESDAY					
THURSDAY					
FRIDAY					
SATURDAY					
SUNDAY					
TOTAL	Strength: number of days _____		Aerobic: number of minutes _____		

Physical Exercise/Activity Log

	DATE	ACTIVITY	DURATION (MINUTES)	AEROBIC OR STRENGTH?	INTENSITY
MONDAY					
TUESDAY					
WEDNESDAY					
THURSDAY					
FRIDAY					
SATURDAY					
SUNDAY					
TOTAL	Strength: number of days		Aerobic: number of minutes		

10,000 Steps Program

If you are currently not getting any physical exercise at all, start by walking. You can incorporate walking into all your other daily activities. Keep walking more and more every day until you are taking 10,000 steps a day. Get a simple pedometer to keep track of how much you are walking. The following worksheet will help you set your goals and get you to 10,000 steps a day. To start this program, you'll need to determine your baseline activity in the first week. Track your steps everyday for a week and log into the chart below.

Week 1: Your Baseline

DATE	DAY	# OF STEPS
	1	
	2	
	3	
	4	
	5	
	6	
	7	
	# DAYS LOGGED:	TOTAL WEEK 1:

New Daily Goal

Take the total steps from week one and divide by the number of days you wore the pedometer. Now add 200 to 500 steps to determine your new daily goal for the next week.

TOTAL WEEK 1:		# DAYS LOGGED:		AVERAGE STEPS/DAY:
	÷		=	
AVERAGE STEPS/DAY:		200 TO 500 STEPS		WEEK 2 DAILY GOAL:
	+		=	

Week 2: Daily Goal _____ Steps a Day

DATE	DAY	# OF STEPS
	1	
	2	
	3	
	4	
	5	
	6	
	7	
	# DAYS LOGGED:	TOTAL WEEK 2:

New Daily Goal

TOTAL WEEK 2:		# DAYS LOGGED:		AVERAGE STEPS/DAY:
	÷		=	
AVERAGE STEPS/DAY:		200 TO 500 STEPS		WEEK 3 DAILY GOAL:
	+		=	

Week 3: Daily Goal _____ Steps a Day

DATE	DAY	# OF STEPS
	1	
	2	
	3	
	4	
	5	
	6	
	7	
	# DAYS LOGGED:	TOTAL WEEK 3:

New Daily Goal

TOTAL WEEK 3:		# DAYS LOGGED:		AVERAGE STEPS/DAY:
	÷		=	
AVERAGE STEPS/DAY:		200 TO 500 STEPS		WEEK 4 DAILY GOAL:
	+		=	

Week 4: Daily Goal _____ Steps a Day

DATE	DAY	# OF STEPS
	1	
	2	
	3	
	4	
	5	
	6	
	7	
	# DAYS LOGGED:	TOTAL WEEK 4:

New Daily Goal

TOTAL WEEK 4:		# DAYS LOGGED:		AVERAGE STEPS/DAY:
	÷		=	
AVERAGE STEPS/DAY:		200 TO 500 STEPS		WEEK 5 DAILY GOAL:
	+		=	

Week 5: Daily Goal _____ Steps a Day

DATE	DAY	# OF STEPS
	1	
	2	
	3	
	4	
	5	
	6	
	7	
	# DAYS LOGGED:	TOTAL WEEK 5:

New Daily Goal

TOTAL WEEK 5:		# DAYS LOGGED:		AVERAGE STEPS/DAY:
	÷		=	
AVERAGE STEPS/DAY:		200 TO 500 STEPS		WEEK 6 DAILY GOAL:
	+		=	

Week 6: Daily Goal _____ Steps a Day

DATE	DAY	# OF STEPS
	1	
	2	
	3	
	4	
	5	
	6	
	7	
	# DAYS LOGGED:	TOTAL WEEK 6:

New Daily Goal

TOTAL WEEK 6:		# DAYS LOGGED:		AVERAGE STEPS/DAY:
	÷		=	
AVERAGE STEPS/DAY:		200 TO 500 STEPS		WEEK 7 DAILY GOAL:
	+		=	

Week 7: Daily Goal _____ Steps a Day

DATE	DAY	# OF STEPS
	1	
	2	
	3	
	4	
	5	
	6	
	7	
	# DAYS LOGGED:	TOTAL WEEK 7:

New Daily Goal

TOTAL WEEK 7:		# DAYS LOGGED:		AVERAGE STEPS/DAY:
	÷		=	
AVERAGE STEPS/DAY:		200 TO 500 STEPS		WEEK 8 DAILY GOAL:
	+		=	

Week 8: Daily Goal _____ Steps a Day

DATE	DAY	# OF STEPS
	1	
	2	
	3	
	4	
	5	
	6	
	7	
	# DAYS LOGGED:	TOTAL WEEK 8:

Self-Evaluation

At the end of each week, reflect on how you did in implementing healthy changes in nutrition and exercise. Write down what you feel you did well and what you could do better. Brainstorm about what you think were barriers to the changes you wanted to make and how to get past those barriers the next week. Congratulate yourself on things you did well and keep them up!

	AREAS OF CHANGE	WHAT I DID WELL	HOW I COULD DO BETTER
WEEK 1	Nutrition		
	Exercise		
WEEK 2	Nutrition		
	Exercise		
WEEK 3	Nutrition		
	Exercise		

	AREAS OF CHANGE	WHAT I DID WELL	HOW I COULD DO BETTER
WEEK 4	Nutrition		
	Exercise		
WEEK 5	Nutrition		
	Exercise		
WEEK 6	Nutrition		
	Exercise		
WEEK 7	Nutrition		
	Exercise		
WEEK 8	Nutrition		
	Exercise		

RESOURCES

Here are some free online resources to help you on your way to a healthier liver:

www.hsph.harvard.edu/nutritionsource
   Set up by the Harvard School of Public Health, this website provides comprehensive diet and nutrition information.

http://hp2010.nhlbihin.net/portion/servingcard7.pdf
   This is a printable pocket guide on ideal portion sizes.

Websites on Nutrition Labels

www.fda.gov/Food/IngredientsPackagingLabeling/LabelingNutrition/ucm274593.htm#see1

www.choosemyplate.gov/downloads/NutritionFactsLabel.pdf

www.heart.org/HEARTORG/GettingHealthy/NutritionCenter/HeartSmartShopping/Reading-Food-Nutrition-Labels_UCM_300132_Article.jsp

www.webmd.com/diet/healthtool-food-calorie-counter
   This website helps you understand the nutrition breakdown of specific foods.

http://nutritiondata.self.com
   This website lets you analyze recipes to see how they measure up

nutritionally. It is useful for when you want to try a new recipe or modify a recipe to be healthier.

www.bidmc.org/YourHealth/BIDMCInteractive/Break-Through-Your-Set-Point.aspx
This free online weight-loss course is offered on Beth Israel Deaconess Medical Center on its website.

www.heart.org/HEARTORG/GettingHealthy/WeightManagement/LosingWeight/Losing-Weight_UCM_307904_Article.jsp
The American Heart Association provides tips on healthy weight loss.

Websites help you plan. Start by setting health and nutrition goals, and then keep track of eating and physical activities to see how you are doing with your goals. Play around on each website to see which site you prefer. Some people find it easier to track on a smartphone app. Some apps, such as MyFitnessPal, have a scan function. If you are at an airport shop looking for a snack, scan the bar codes of the different packages for instant nutritional information to help you make a smarter choice.

Most people find it hard to enter their food and activities over the long term. Stick with it for at least 2 weeks to get a sense of how you are faring in your goals. Knowledge is power. Arming yourself with knowledge about your dietary and physical activity habits will give you the power to change. These resources will also help you during holidays or travel when sticking to your routine is tougher.

www.supertracker.usda.gov/default.aspx

www.myfitnesspal.com
This is also a free smartphone and tablet application.

www.webmd.com/diet/food-fitness-planner

www.healthydiningfinder.com
For eating out, this website provides you some healthy choice menu items for selected restaurant chains. A team of registered dietitians has

analyzed menus and chosen some items that meet their criteria for healthy choices. Read their criteria so you understand how they make their choices.

Useful Smartphone and Tablet Apps

Here are some smartphone apps to help set personal nutrition and fitness goals and track your foods and physical activities.

Calorie Counter and Diet Tracker by Calorie Count (on iPhone)

Calorie Counter and Diet Tracker HD (on iPad)

Calorie Counter (on Android)

Calorie Counter & Diet Tracker by MyFitnessPal (on iPhone, iPad, and Android)

Lose it! Weight Loss Program and Calorie Counter (on iPhone, tablets and Android)

Fast Food Calorie Counter by Mobigloo (on iPhone and Blackberry)

FitDay (iPhone and iPad)

Fooducate (iPhone, iPad, and Android)

Smartphone Running Apps

These apps use the GPS in your phone to help track your distance, speed, pace, and calories burned. Some link to your music playlist so you can enjoy your favorite music while running.

Nike running app (iPhone and iPad)

Map My Run (iPhone, Android, and Blackberry)

Run Keeper (iPhone and Android)

Other Helpful Apps

GateGuru lists dining choices near an airport gate so you can make more informed decisions.

Locavore tells you which fruits and vegetables are at peak freshness at your location and provides a map of the closest farmer's market.

Good Food Near You lists healthy choices at nearby eateries.

INDEX

ACKNOWLEDGMENTS

I would like to thank the following people without whose support this book would not have been possible:

My husband, Ted, whose unconditional support carried me through all the lows and highs over the years. He has the ability to always make me laugh–proving that laughter sometimes is the best medicine.

My parents, who have always sacrificed their own interests to provide us with every opportunity in life. Their support has continued throughout my whole life, including the endless hours of babysitting so that I could get the book done. Wonderful parents do make the most wonderful (albeit more permissive) grandparents.

Amami and Agong, the best grandparents, whose words of encouragement are still with me even though they are not.

My older brothers, Dave and Jerry, for toughening me up while growing up. My sisters-in-law, Jen and Roselle, for softening them up.

My mother-in-law, Hana, for the time and love she has showered on Sammi as well so I can finish the book.

My aunts and uncles who taught me the joys of family and sharing food.

My patients, the inspiration for this book.

My coauthor, Asha, whose friendship and collaboration means the world to me.

Our editor, Alice, book agent, Dalyn, and publisher for helping to make this book a reality.

—Michelle

Thank you to my colleagues, mentors, and patients at Beth Israel Deaconess Medical Center who have always inspired me to work hard and be a better educator! This is the place that helped me grow professionally and will always have a special place in my heart. Boston Strong!

My coauthor Michelle for asking me to go on this adventure with her—we did it!

Our editor Alice for her dedication to make sure the book is perfect, and everyone at Hollan and Ulysses Press for making this a reality!

My parents who have always sacrificed so much in their lives so that my brother and I could have everything we needed. As physicians themselves, my parents set an example to be compassionate, kind, and generous with their time and knowledge with everyone, especially to people with ill health. My mother has always motivated me to be the best in everything I do, and I will forever be grateful to her for instilling this in me from a young age. She wanted me to follow my dreams and this book is certainly one of them.

My brother for his comic relief no matter how tough things were—he always manages to make me laugh!

Finally my husband, Sumeet, who is my biggest supporter! A lot of the writing was done at night, on weekends and holidays, and times that were inconvenient to my family. Without his patience, encouragement, and support this wouldn't have been possible! I look up to him every day and he teaches me to be a better person in so many ways.

My entire family including my in-laws and close friends who were always encouraging me to accomplish this book even though it took my time away from them!

—Asha

ABOUT THE AUTHORS

Michelle Lai, MD, MPH is a hepatologist at Beth Israel Deaconess Medical Center, one of the top liver health centers in the country, and an assistant professor in medicine at Harvard Medical School. She takes care of patients with liver diseases and is working on clinical research in non-alcoholic fatty liver disease. Michelle has published articles on viral hepatitis, liver cirrhosis, liver transplantation, non-alcoholic fatty liver disease, and noninvasive evaluation of liver diseases. She earned a bachelor of arts degree in biology from Harvard University, and a medical degree and a master's degree in public health from Columbia University. She completed her internal medicine, gastroenterology, and transplant hepatology training at Beth Israel Deaconess Medical Center.

Asha R. Kasaraneni, MSc, RD, LDN, CNSC is a dietitian at the Transplant Institute at Beth Deaconess Medical Center in Boston. She provides dietary recommendations to liver, kidney, and pancreas patients both pre- and post-transplant. Asha earned a bachelor of science degree from Leeds Metropolitan University, England, and a master's degree from Northumbria University, England, and later attended Simmons College in Boston. She completed her dietetic internship at Beth Israel Deaconess Medical Center. In addition to being a registered dietitian, she is licensed as a certified nutrition support clinician, a credential awarded by ASPEN (American Society for Parenteral and Enteral Nutrition). Asha and Michelle have been colleagues and friends for years, and share a passion for cooking.